CASE STUDIES IN DENTAL HYGIENE

Evelyn M. Thomson, BSDH, MS
Senior Lecturer
Gene W. Hirschfeld School of Dental Hygiene
Old Dominion University
Norfolk, Virginia

Deborah Blythe Bauman, BSDH, MS
Associate Professor
Gene W. Hirschfeld School of Dental Hygiene
Old Dominion University
Norfolk, Virginia

Deanne Shuman, BSDH, MS, PhD
Professor and Chair
Gene W. Hirschfeld School of Dental Hygiene
Old Dominion University
Norfolk, Virginia

Esther K. Andrews, CDA, RDA, RDH, MA
Private Practice Dental Hygienist
Chicago, Illinois

Prentice Hall

Upper Saddle River, New Jersey 07458

Library of Congress Cataloging-in-Publication Data
Case studies in dental hygiene / Evelyn M. Thomson . . . [et al.].
     p. ; cm.
Includes bibliograhical references.
     ISBN 0-13-018571-X
     1. Dental hygiene. 2. Dental hygiene—Case studies. 3. Dental
hygiene—Examinations, questions, etc.
     [DNLM: 1. Dental Care—methods—Case Report. 2. Dental
Care—methods—Examination Questions. 3. Dental Hygienists—Case
Report. 4. Dental Hygienists—Examination Questions. 5. Dental
Prophylaxis—methods—Case Report. 6. Dental Prophylaxis—
methods—Examination Questions. 7. Oral Health—Case Report. 8.
Oral Health—Examination Questions. 9. Radiography,
Dental—methods—Case Report. 10. Radiography, Dental—
methods—Examination Questions. WU 18.2 C337 2003] I. Thomson,
Evelyn M.
     RK60.5 .C365 2003
     617.6′01—dc21   2002002216

Publisher: *Julie Levin Alexander*
Publisher's Assistant: *Regina Bruno*
Senior Acquisitions Editor: *Mark Cohen*
Assistant Editor: *Melissa Kerian*
Editoral Assistant: *Mary Ellen Ruitenberg*
Director of Production and Manufacturing: *Bruce Johnson*
Managing Editor for Production: *Patrick Walsh*
Production Liaison: *Alexander Ivchenko*
Production Editor: *Jessica Balch (Pine Tree Compositon)*
Manufacturing Manager: *Ilene Sanford*
Manufacturing Buyer: *Pat Brown*
Creative Director: *Cheryl Asherman*
Cover Design Coordinator: *Maria Guglielmo-Walsh*
Formatting: *Pine Tree Composition*
Marketing Manager: *Nicole Benson*
Product Information Manager: *Rachele Triano*
Printer/Binder: *Banta Harrisonburg*
Copyeditor: *Joseph Pomerance*
Cover Design: *Joseph DePinho*
Cover Printer: *Phoenix Color*

Pearson Education Ltd., London
Pearson Education Australia Pty. Limited, Sydney
Pearson Education Singapore, Pte. Ltd.
Pearson Education North Asia Ltd., Hong Kong
Pearson Education Canada, Ltd., Toronto
Pearson Educación de Mexico, S.A. de C.V.
Pearson Education—Japan, Tokyo
Pearson Education Malaysia, Pte. Ltd.
Pearson Education, Upper Saddle River, New Jersey

Notice: Care has been taken to confirm the accuracy of the information presented in this book. The authors, editors, and the publisher, however, cannot accept any responsibility for errors or omissions or for the consequences for application of the information in this book and make no warranty, express or implied, with respect to its contents.

The authors and the publisher have exerted every effort to ensure that drug selections and dosages set forth in this text are in accord with current recommendations and practice at time of publication. However, in view of ongoing research, changes in government regulations, and the constant flow of information relating to drug therapy and drug reactions, the reader is urged to check the package inserts of all drugs for any change in indications of dosage and for added warnings and precautions. This is particularly important when the recommended agent is a new and/or infrequently employed drug.

The authors and publisher disclaim all responsibility for any liability, loss, injury, or damage incurred as a consequence, directly or indirectly, of the use and application of any of the contents of this volume.

10 9 8 7 6 5
ISBN 0-13-018571-X

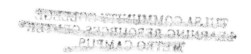

Contents

Preface

Educators need case-based learning tools that may be integrated throughout the dental hygiene curriculum. Within the educational environment exists the goal to assist students in linking basic knowledge to dental hygiene care that is evidence-based and client-centered. With the constantly evolving knowledge base and changing technologies, dental hygiene faculty are challenged to incorporate educational technologies that exceed knowledge acquisition and focus on critical decision making. *Case Studies in Dental Hygiene* is a viable educational tool to help students learn to apply basic knowledge to client care and to prepare them for success on national, regional and state examinations which have a client care focus.

Case Studies in Dental Hygiene is designed to guide the development of critical thinking skills and the application of theory to care at all levels of dental hygiene education—from beginning to advanced students. Additionally, during the course of their formal education, dental hygiene students can be exposed only to a small spectrum of cases they might encounter in the real world. The diversity of the cases in this text provides an avenue for simulating experiences students might not encounter in their education. This text is designed to cover a broad array of topics, to be adaptable for use in a variety of courses, and to be used across student knowledge and skill levels.

This text is designed to be utilized throughout the dental hygiene curriculum. Because the questions and decisions regarding treatment of each case span the dental hygiene sciences and clinical practice protocols, this text will find a place in enhancing each and every course required of dental hygiene students. It is expected that *Case Studies in Dental Hygiene* would be introduced at the beginning of the student's educational experience and be utilized throughout the program of study. As the students' knowledge base develops, the answers to the more complex questions would become apparent. If the text were introduced early in the program, students would realize the link between theory and client care immediately. Once exposed to the cases, students progress through the program with a heightened awareness, a "need to know," as new material is introduced which can be applied to answer case-based questions. Additionally, *Case Studies in Dental Hygiene* makes an excellent review text for graduating dental hygiene students preparing to take the Dental Hygiene National Board Examination.

Case Studies in Dental Hygiene presents oral health case situations representing a variety of clients that would typically be encountered in clinical settings. There are 10 cases, 2 each representing the following client types: pediatric, adult periodontally involved, geriatric, special needs, and medically compromised. Each case contains a medical history, dental history, vital signs (including blood pressure, pulse, and respiratory rates), radiographs, dental and periodontal charting, intraoral photographs, and

v

photographs of study models, where applicable. Additionally, learning objectives and multiple-choice questions are identified for each case. Questions are subdivided into the following categories: assessing client characteristics, obtaining and interpreting dental radiographs, planning and managing dental hygiene care; performing periodontal procedures, using preventive agents, and providing supportive treatment services. Each question is clearly identified as "basic" or "complex," further guiding educators and students to use each case to maximum benefit. Students will be challenged to seek answers and select appropriate care for the clients in each case scenario. Correct answers and rationales for incorrect responses are provided for all questions. Providing descriptive rationales for incorrect answers further enhances learning. Reflective activities and a section incorporating the Human Needs Conceptual Model to Dental Hygiene Practice guide the instructor in developing additional learning activities for the student. The rapidly increasing, constantly changing knowledge base and technologies associated with clinical practice mandate that dental hygiene professionals be prepared to provide oral care that meets the needs of the whole client. The Human Needs Conceptual Model to Dental Hygiene Practice has been established as a means of linking oral care with the general health of an individual. Although many dental hygiene programs have incorporated the Human Needs Conceptual Model into their curriculum, others are in need of educational tools which assist with this incorporation. *Case Studies in Dental Hygiene* provides educators with a bank of ready-made cases with which to guide students to integrate client needs or deficits with dental hygiene care planning. Each case lists suggestions for creating decision-making opportunities for the students, regarding client care and treatment recommendations that promote oral health and prevent oral diseases.

HOW TO USE THIS BOOK

Each chapter contains one case scenario, making it a stand-alone module that may be introduced in any order and at any time during the curriculum. While there are a variety of ways in which to utilize the case studies, educators may benefit from the suggestions listed here. Cases C and D, The Periodontally Involved Adult Client, could be used as required reading for the preclinical student to introduce the dental hygiene process of care. Because each case contains questions that are knowledge-based as well as complex decision-making questions, the beginning student may be directed to answer the "basic" questions. During theory class, a discussion of these answers may help to increase the incidence of critical thinking skills and can reinforce and facilitate learning in a dynamic, stimulating manner motivating the student to more fully participate in the learning process. Because the questions for each case are subdivided into client assessment, radiographic services, planning and management of care, periodontal procedures, and supplemental services, instructors of basic dental hygiene sciences may easily identify those questions which supplement learning in their disciplines. The radiology instructor may utilize the "basic" questions of all the cases, directing the beginning student to those questions under the subdivision "obtaining and interpreting dental radiographs" while the pharmacology instructor may use Cases I and J, The Medically Compromised Client, to provide a realistic setting to assist students in linking drug interactions which may contraindicate dental hygiene care with planning and managing treatment. Cases A and B, The Pediatric Client, may provide an opportunity for the student to identify eruption patterns, learned in head and neck anatomy or tooth and root morphology courses. Applying theory and knowledge gained in the basic dental hygiene sciences to solve problems encountered through case-based questioning allows the student to become actively involved in the learning process. After all, the challenge of case-based instruction is to maximize students' synthesis of theoretical material and provide a link between science, theory, and clinical practice. *Case Studies in Dental Hygiene* may compliment and enhance material learned in other texts. For example, students learning instrument design from a theory book may link application of this knowledge when challenged by case photographs and charts to choose an appropriate instrument for scaling a specific area. Radiographic problem solving skills are further enhanced by examination of the case radiographs when the student is challenged not only to identify technique and processing errors, but also to recommend corrective action.

In addition to basic questions, each case contains complex questions that challenge advanced students to develop improved clinical reasoning that will assist them in real-world clinical practice. As students progress through the curriculum, the same cases may be revisited through the use of complex questions. Students usually respond favorably to the opportunity to apply knowledge gained in the classroom to fictional cases. The ability to plan treatment and simulate implementation through case study provides the student with a stress-free environment in which to make decisions. Students report increased confidence when faced with treatment planning and implementation decisions regarding clients in the clinical setting. Students also perceive an increase in confidence regarding preparation for national and regional board examinations when they have been given the opportunity to practice decision making.

In case-based teaching, a frequent faculty complaint is that students and faculty have difficulty integrating information from various courses within the discipline to the case-based format. Healthcare educators are fully cognizant that effective clinical judgment only comes from experience, since it is the use of real life situations which encourages student analysis and decision making in areas relevant to professional practice. However, most faculty do not consider themselves experts on all dimensions of a problem, and as a result may be limited in their use of case studies. To overcome the limited use of case studies to specific disciplines, *Case Studies in Dental Hygiene* was written by several authors, each an expert in a specific aspect of dental hygiene care. This multi-author approach to the development of the cases contained in this book, is intended to provide other dental hygiene educators with a ready-made bank of cases upon which to build meaningful learning activities for the student. Additionally, the authors hope that the format and content of *Case Studies in Dental Hygiene* will provide students with an opportunity to practice critical decision-making skills and reinforce and facilitate learning in a dynamic, stimulating manner, thereby motivating students to more fully participate in the learning process. This book was designed specifically to encourage dental hygiene students to base client care decisions on knowledge gained in theory, thus fostering in students an appreciation of the link between theory and clinical practice.

Acknowledgments

Case Studies in Dental Hygiene represents a collection of teaching cases developed over years of clinical dental hygiene instruction and interaction with colleagues. This book would not have been possible, without the support and assistance of the students, faculty and staff at Old Dominion University's Gene W. Hirschfeld School of Dental Hygiene. The authors are particularly grateful to those students who recognized challenging case clients, and were able to share their learning experiences, and to the clients who consented to donate personal data to be part of this book.

The photography and radiographic representations of the cases would not have been possible without the cooperation and efforts of the following Old Dominion University dental hygiene students: Jennifer Caswell, Shane Davis, Nicole Fisher, Carrie Hammer, Lisa Kelly, Julie Tebault, and Jolyn Wurm. Additionally, a special thanks goes to Virginia Beach orthodontist Lawrence A. Klar, DDS, MS, for his photographic contribution.

The authors wish to acknowledge the following individuals for their professional contributions and expert feedback: in the area of periodontology, Lynn Tolle, BSDH, MS, Professor, Old Dominion University, and in the area of geriatric dentistry, Lynnette M. Engeswick, RDH, MS, Assistant Professor, Minnesota State University.

A very special thank-you goes to our families and friends whose contributions of time and support are greatly appreciated, particularly Mike Thomson and Brian Steele, whose volunteer efforts contributed to case development; Laurie Semple for her encouragement; and in remembrance of Robert L. Newton.

Finally, the authors would like to express appreciation to Mark Cohen, Senior Editor, Prentice Hall Health, for his guidance and patience throughout the process and to Melissa Kerian, Assistant Editor, Prentice Hall Health, for her assistance in the final stages of production.

Evelyn Thomson
Debbie Bauman
Deanne Shuman
Esther Andrews

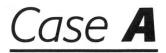

Case **A**

Pediatric Client
Maya Patel

Learning Goals

Following integration of core scientific concepts and application of dental hygiene theory to the care of this client, the student will be able to

1. **Assess client characteristics.**
   A. Identify developmental normalities and abnormalities of the dentition.
   B. Recognize oral conditions of the tongue.
   C. Identify normal vital signs in the pediatric client.
   D. Recognize the signs of anxiety in the pediatric client.
   E. Identify side effects of medications used to treat asthma.
   F. Identify side effects of medications used to treat allergies.

2. **Obtain and interpret dental radiographs.**
   A. Determine the recommended oral radiographic projection for a pediatric client.
   B. Identify anatomic structures radiographically.
   C. Recognize the cause of radiographic image distortion.

3. **Plan and manage dental hygiene care.**
   A. Individualize oral health care instructions for the pediatric client.
   B. Apply concept of selective stain removal.
   C. Recognize the signs of an emergency situation and initiate appropriate management actions.
   D. Appropriately manage the pediatric client for successful completion of treatment.

4. **Perform periodontal procedures.**
   A. Recognize microorganisms associated with gingivitis.
   B. Select the most appropriate instruments for subgingival deplaquing for the periodontally healthy pediatric client.

5. **Use preventive agents**
   A. Select teeth for sealant placement.
   B. Evaluate the benefits of personal mechanical oral hygiene care for dental caries control.
   C. Select professionally applied topical fluoride treatment for the client's needs.

6. **Provide supportive treatment services**
   A. Demonstrate knowledge of impression-taking procedure.
   B. Identify nutritional data critical to oral health.

> ### *Situation*
>
> Maya Patel's mother brought her to the dental office today for a checkup. When asked, her mother admits that Maya's last appointment was "more than 6 months ago." Maya appears unnaturally stiff and short of breath as she quickly answers questions about her oral health. She appears overly willing to cooperate and is opening and closing a poetry journal she has brought with her.
>
> *For a detailed client history, including radiographs and color photos, see pages I-2 to I-5.*

CLIENT'S HUMAN NEEDS DEFICITS

Because the client's oral wellness is interrelated with the client's attitudes toward health, values, and practices, and with family and cultural influences, it is important that the dental hygiene care plan be client-centered. Examination of human needs to assist the client in developing and maintaining appropriate self-care revealed the following deficits:

1. Protection from health risks

   Due to: Risk for an asthma attack

   Evidenced by: Potential for a medical emergency

2. Responsibility for oral health

   Due to: Lack of regular oral care by parents, inadequate oral health behaviors and parental supervision

   Evidenced by: Gingivitis and caries

3. Skin and mucous membrane integrity of the head and neck

   Due to: Plaque bacteria and inadequate oral health behaviors

   Evidenced by: The presence of gingival inflammation and bleeding

4. Biologically sound dentition

   Due to: Future caries risk

   Evidenced by: Existing carious lesion

5. Freedom from anxiety and stress

   Due to: Fear related to dental treatment

   Evidenced by: Client report and anxious behaviors

QUESTIONS

Basic Questions in Assessing Client Characteristics

1. The anterior teeth exhibit which of the following conditions?
   A. Perikymata
   B. Hypoplasia
   C. Fluorosis
   D. Mamelons
   E. Attrition

2. Which of the following is the correct assessment of the appearance of this client's tongue?

   A. Lymphangioma
   B. Fissured
   C. Coated
   D. Macroglossia
   E. Ulcerated

3. The raised, white object that appears between the mandibular left permanent canine and the mandibular left primary second molar is MOST LIKELY

   A. Mandibular tori.
   B. Retained primary root tip.
   C. Erupting permanent premolar.
   D. Aphthous ulcer.
   E. Developmental cyst.

4. Which of the following best describes this client's vital signs?

   A. Respiration rate is considered high.
   B. Respiration rate is considered low.
   C. Pulse rate is considered high.
   D. Pulse rate is considered within normal range.
   E. Blood pressure is considered high.

Complex Questions in Assessing Client Characteristics

5. This client's behavior today may be clinical signs of all of the following EXCEPT one. Which is the EXCEPTION?

   A. Asthma attack onset
   B. Arrested cognitive development
   C. Moderate anxiety
   D. Medication side effects
   E. Emotional disorder

6. All of the following are associated side effects of this client's medications EXCEPT one. Which is the EXCEPTION?

   A. Xerostomia
   B. Taste changes
   C. Increased anxiety
   D. Sore throat
   E. Gingival bleeding

Basic Questions in Obtaining and Interpreting Dental Radiographs

7. What is the name of the anatomic structure seen as a horizontal radiopacity above the maxillary teeth, marked by the arrow, in the panoramic radiograph?

   A. Incisive foramen
   B. Median palatine suture
   C. Nasal fossae
   D. Nasal septum
   E. Hard palate

Complex Questions in Obtaining and Interpreting Dental Radiographs

8. Which of the following is the BEST reason why the panoramic radiograph was chosen over intraoral radiographs for this client?
    A. Possibility of asthma attack
    B. Patient must remain in an upright position
    C. Exaggerated gag reflex
    D. Lower radiation dosage

9. What is the reason for the shortened appearance of the mandibular incisors on the panoramic radiograph?
    A. Teeth tipped out of the focal trough
    B. External physiologic resorption
    C. Apices have not fully formed
    D. Microdontia of the central and lateral incisors

Basic Questions in Planning and Managing Dental Hygiene Care

10. What method of tongue debridement is recommended for this client?
    A. Brush the tongue with a toothbrush.
    B. Scrape the tongue with a tongue scraper.
    C. Rinse the mouth daily with an oxygenating mouth rinse.
    D. Irrigate the tongue with an oral irrigator.
    E. Have the patient suck on a breath freshener tablet.

11. Which of the following is the method of choice for extrinsic stain removal for this client?
    A. Rubber cup coronal polishing
    B. Air-powder abrasive system
    C. Scaling and toothbrush prophylaxis
    D. Toothbrushing with commercial prophylaxis paste
    E. Ultrasonic scaling for stain removal

Complex Questions in Planning and Managing Dental Hygiene Care

12. Approximately halfway through the dental appointment, this client complains of trouble breathing. The clinician should do all of the following EXCEPT one. Which is the EXCEPTION?
    A. Continue conversation that calms the client.
    B. Terminate the dental procedure at once.
    C. Remove all instruments from the client's mouth.
    D. Place the client in the Trendelenberg position.
    E. Administer a bronchodilator.

13. What method of client management would BEST serve this client?
    A. Tell, show, do
    B. Oral sedation
    C. Papoose board restriction
    D. Hypnosis
    E. Biofeedback

Basic Questions in Performing Periodontal Procedures

14. Which of the following microorganisms are associated with this client's periodontal disease state?
    A. *Streptococcus salivaris*
    B. *Fusobacterium nucleatum* and *Prevotella intermedia*
    C. Actinomyces, Streptococcus, and Fusobacterium
    D. *Streptococcus mutans* and lactobaccilli
    E. *Actinobacillus actinomycetemcomitans*

15. Which of the following would be the best instrument for subgingival deplaquing in this client's case?
    A. Anterior sickle scaler
    B. Universal sickle scaler
    C. Area-specific Gracey curets
    D. Universal curet
    E. Ultrasonic scaling device

Basic Questions in Using Preventive Agents

16. Which of this client's teeth are indicated for sealants?
    A. Primary first molars
    B. Primary second molars
    C. Permanent first premolars
    D. Permanent first molars
    E. Permanent second molars

Complex Questions in Using Preventive Agents

17. Which of the following preventive agents is indicated for this client?
    A. Interproximal brush
    B. Fluoride rinse
    C. Tartar control toothpaste
    D. Oral irrigator
    E. Chlorohexidine gluconate

18. Which of the following professionally applied topical fluorides is the method of choice for this client?
    A. Acidulated phosphate fluoride
    B. Neutral sodium fluoride
    C. Stannous fluoride
    D. Sodium monofluorophosphate fluoride

Basic Questions in Providing Supportive Treatment Services

19. All of the following are considered critical to nutritional counseling for this client EXCEPT one. Which is the EXCEPTION?
    A. Cultural food preferences
    B. Inclusion of person responsible for meal preparation
    C. Medications interference with metabolism
    D. Frequency of carbohydrate intake
    E. Number of servings from food groups

20. Which of the following is the MOST LIKELY cause of difficulty for taking impressions on this client?
    A. Sensitive gingiva
    B. Tight frenum attachment
    C. Exaggerated gag reflex
    D. Occlusal open bite

Answers appear on pages 71–73.

Reflective Activities

1. People from India who practice the Hindu religion consider cows sacred and do not eat beef. Review the nutrients available from the consumption of beef and recommend other nutritional sources for these nutrients to improve oral health.

2. Examine the ethnic, cultural, or regional dietary practices and/or problems present in the population in your area. Plan a 3-day menu that would fulfill the recommended dietary allowance and incorporate food preferences for this population.

3. Discuss preappointment dental hygiene interventions that will create a child-centered, nonthreatening environment to minimize this client's anxiety.

REFERENCES

Bouffard C: Controlling pain and anxiety. *Access* (13)4, 14–18, 1999.

Casamassimo PS, Griffiths P, Nowak A: Anticipatory guidance in dentistry. *Dental Hygienist News* (2)5, 19–21, 1989.

Darby ML, Walsh MM: *Dental Hygiene Theory and Practice.* Philadelphia: Saunders, 1994, pp. 248–249, 343, 354–357.

Davis JR, Stegeman CA: *The Dental Hygienist's Guide to Nutritional Care,* Philadelphia: Saunders, 1998, pp. 363–378.

Gage T, Pickett F: *Mosby's Dental Drug Reference,* 5th ed. St. Louis: Mosby, 2001, pp. 28–29, 390.

Haring JI, Jansen L: *Dental Radiography Principles and Techniques,* 2nd ed. Philadelphia: Saunders, 2000, pp. 357–359.

Malamed SF: *Medical Emergencies in the Dental Office,* 5th ed. St. Louis: Mosby, 2000, pp. 36, 39–49, 214–221.

Miller RL, Gould AR, Bernstein ML, Read CJ: *General and Oral Pathology for the Dental Hygienist.* St. Louis: Mosby, 1995, pp. 179–183.

Oral B: *Comparison of Fluorides.* Braun Oral-B Consumer Services, 1 Gillette Park, South Boston, MA, 1999.

Perry DA, Beemsterboer P, Taggart EJ: *Periodontology for the Dental Hygienist,* 2nd ed. Philadelphia: Saunders, 2001, pp. 53–68.

Pinkham JR: *Pediatric Dentistry: Infancy Through Adolescence.* Philadelphia: WB Saunders, 1988, pp. 239–245, 271–272, 342–343.

Slots J, Taubman M: *Contemporary Oral Microbiology and Immunology.* St. Louis: Mosby, 1993, p. 429.

Wilkins EM: *Clinical Practice of the Dental Hygienist,* 8th ed. Philadelphia: Lippincott Williams & Wilkins, 1999, pp. 110, 173, 346–347, 365, 441–479, 482, 603, 607.

Winkler MW, Deschepper EJ, Dean JA, Moore BK, Cochran MA, Ewoldsen N: Using a resin modified glass ionomer as an occlusal sealant: A one-year clinical study. *Journal of the American Dental Association,* (127)10, 1508–1514.

Woelful J: *Dental Anatomy and Its Relevance to Dentistry,* 4th ed. Philadelphia: Lea & Febiger, 1990, pp. 100, 114.

Learning Goals

Following integration of core scientific concepts and application of dental hygiene theory to the care of this client, the student will be able to

1. **Assess client characteristics.**
   A. Classify the facial profile.
   B. Classify occlusion using Angle's system of malocclusion.
   C. Recognize eruption/exfoliation patterns.
   D. Recall the reason for nocturnal bruxism.
   E. Recognize the need for orthodontic evaluation.
   F. Differentiate dental fluorosis from other white spot lesions.

2. **Obtain and interpret dental radiographs.**
   A. Identify oral conditions indicating the need for a cephalometric radiograph.
   B. Interpret radiopaque artifacts commonly present in a cephalometric radiograph.
   C. Differentiate between normal radiographic anatomy and pathosis.

3. **Plan and manage dental hygiene care.**
   A. Plan oral health instruction for an adolescent using spit tobacco.
   B. Plan individualized dental hygiene care for adolescent clients.
   C. Recognize the cognitive development stages of adolescent clients.
   D. Choose oral self-care methods based on individual needs of the client.
   E. Plan individualized oral hygiene instruction.
   F. Apply dental hygiene interventions to help prevent nicotine addiction in adolescents.
   G. Recognize ways in which the dental hygienist can educate youth on the oral implications of developing a tobacco use habit.

4. **Perform periodontal procedures.**
   A. Describe gingival appearance.
   B. Identify the causes of gingival inflammation.

5. **Use preventive agents.**
   A. Select the appropriate extrinsic stain removal procedure based on client assessment.

6. **Provide supportive treatment services.**
   A. Identify the need for mouthguard protection.

> ### *Situation*
>
> *Zack Ware is a physically active sixth-grader who spends his free time playing baseball and skateboarding with friends. Although he knows that spit tobacco is not a safe alternative to smoking, his peers have suggested that professional athletes benefit from its use.*
>
> *For a detailed client history, including radiographs and color photos, see pages I-6 to I-9.*

CLIENT'S HUMAN NEEDS DEFICITS

Because the client's oral wellness is interrelated with the client's attitudes toward health, values, and practices, and with family and cultural influences, it is important that the dental hygiene care plan be client-centered. Examination of human needs to assist the client in developing and maintaining appropriate self-care revealed the following deficits:

1. Protection from health risks

   Due to: Increased risk for oral injury
   Evidenced by: Self-reported skateboarding

   Due to: Increased risk for oral lesions
   Evidenced by: Self-reported spit tobacco use

2. Responsibility for oral health

   Due to: Inadequate oral health behaviors and parental supervision
   Evidenced by: Gingivitis and dental caries

3. Skin and mucous membrane integrity of the head and neck

   Due to: Bacterial plaque and inadequate oral health behaviors
   Evidenced by: The presence of gingival inflammation and bleeding

4. Biologically sound dentition

   Due to: Future caries risk
   Evidenced by: Existing carious lesion

QUESTIONS

Basic Questions in Assessing Client Characteristics

1. Which of the following terms best describe this client's facial profile?
   A. Mesognathic
   B. Prognathic
   C. Retrognathic
   D. Orthognatic

2. What is Angle's classification of malocclusion for this client?
   A. Class I
   B. Class II, Division I
   C. Class II, Division II
   D. Class III

3. The primary mandibular left second molar is the next tooth to be exfoliated. The permanent mandibular left second premolar will erupt into this position.

    A. The first statement is true. The second statement is false.
    B. The first statement is false. The second statement is true.
    C. Both statements are true.
    D. Both statements are false.

Complex Questions in Assessing Client Characteristics

4. Which of the following would be considered the MOST LIKELY evidence of the nocturnal bruxism in this client reported by his mother?

    A. Widening of the periodontal ligament spaces
    B. Moderate wear of the primary canines
    C. Temporomandibular joint pain
    D. Occlusal interferences
    E. Genetic predisposition

5. All of this client's permanent teeth are developing normally AND the arch space is adequate for the eruption of his permanent teeth.

    A. The first part of the statement is correct. The second part is incorrect.
    B. The first part of the statement is incorrect. The second part is correct.
    C. Both parts of the statement are correct.
    D. Both parts of the statement are incorrect.

6. The MOST LIKELY assessment of the white spots observed on the anterior teeth of this client is?

    A. Caries
    B. Remineralization
    C. Abrasion
    D. Fluorosis
    E. Wear facets

Basic Questions in Obtaining and Interpreting Dental Radiographs

7. The radiopacities on the permanent mandibular first molars, visible on the panoramic radiograph, are MOST LIKELY which of the following?

    A. Carious lesions
    B. Enamel pearls
    C. Processor artifacts
    D. Orthodontic brackets
    E. Amalgam restorations

8. The cephalometric radiograph was exposed on this client to assess which one of the following?

    A. Growth and development
    B. Periodontal status
    C. Presence of caries
    D. Sinus cavity congestion
    E. Detection of precancerous lesions

Complex Questions in Obtaining and Interpreting Dental Radiographs

9. The radiopaque circle-shaped object that appears on the cephalometric radiograph near the external auditory meatus is MOST LIKELY which one of the following?

    A. Metal earring
    B. Orthodontic band
    C. Cephalostat ear rod
    D. Fixer contamination
    E. Film label

10. The purpose of the radiopaque object visible at the client's nasion on the cephalometric radiograph is to align the

    A. Midsaggital plane.
    B. Frankfort plane.
    C. Occlusal plane.
    D. Vertical plane.
    E. Mandibular plane.

11. Which of the following is the MOST LIKELY reason for the widened appearance of the pulp chambers of the mandibular canines visible on the panoramic radiograph?

    A. Internal resorption
    B. External resorption
    C. Cervical burnout
    D. Incomplete root formation
    E. Nocturnal bruxism

Basic Questions in Planning and Managing Dental Hygiene Care

12. All of the following are true regarding this client's impression of spit tobacco EXCEPT one. Which is the EXCEPTION?

    A. Spit tobacco is highly addictive.
    B. Spit tobacco contains nicotine.
    C. Spit tobacco helps athletic performance.
    D. Spit tobacco is not a safe alternative to cigarettes.

13. Which of the following would be the BEST recommendation for oral self-care for this client?

    A. Automatic toothbrush
    B. Oral irrigation device
    C. Floss threader
    D. Sulcus brush

14. This client is too young to be queried about his tobacco use. Adolescents may experiment with tobacco use due to insecurity, rebelliousness, and identification with role models.

    A. The first statement is true. The second statement is false.
    B. The first statement is false. The second statement is true.
    C. Both statements are true.
    D. Both statements are false.

Complex Questions in Planning and Managing Dental Hygiene Care

15. Which of the following characteristics of development is relevant to this client's age group and managing his preventive oral health self-care instruction?

   A. Incomplete development of a sense of logic will limit an explanation of the disease process.
   B. Continued dependence upon his mother will necessitate parental influence to achieve optimal oral health self-care.
   C. A heightened sense of imagination may increase anxiety related to his lack of adequate self-care behaviors.
   D. Orientation to future possibilities will enhance acceptance of preventive regimens discussed today.
   E. An overriding sense of invincibility will promote a lack of concern for developing good oral health care habits now.

16. Which of the following paired actions will most likely result in an increase in successful oral health education for this client?

   A. Consult his mother to complete a dental history and determine her role in his oral home self-care.
   B. Assess this client's oral conditions and document oral problems to show him a visual representation of his oral health.
   C. Investigate his personal interests to determine what motivates him and present him with a new oral hygiene aid.
   D. Determine his current self-care regime and suggest he increase the time spent performing self-care techniques.

Basic Questions in Performing Periodontal Procedures

17. Which of the following terms BEST describes the appearance of the maxillary facial gingiva prior to orthodontic intervention?

   A. Knifelike
   B. Festooning
   C. Cratering
   D. Clefting
   E. Blunted

Complex Questions in Performing Periodontal Procedures

18. Which of the following is the MOST LIKELY explanation of the appearance of the maxillary facial gingiva prior to orthodontic intervention?

   A. Eruption gingivitis
   B. Malpositioned teeth
   C. Spit tobacco use
   D. Mouth breathing
   E. Bacterial plaque

Basic Questions in Using Preventive Agents

19. Which of the following extrinsic stain removal procedures is indicated for this client?
    A. Rubber cup polishing
    B. Manual toothbrushing
    C. Air-powder abrasive cleaning
    D. Porte polishing

Basic Questions in Providing Supportive Treatment Services

20. A hard plastic thermoset resin mouthguard is indicated for this client BECAUSE skateboarding increases his risk of oral injury.
    A. Both the statement and reason are correct and related.
    B. Both the statement and reason are correct but not related.
    C. The statement is correct but the reason is not.
    D. The statement is not correct but the reason is accurate.
    E. Neither the statement nor reason is correct.

Answers appear on pages 73–76.

Reflective Activities

1. Divide into small groups of three to five students. Each group should list one client-centered goal for each dental hygiene diagnosis for this client. Compile the goals as a group and report to the class. Goals may be written for the cognitive, psychomotor or affective domains or for oral health status improvement. Each goal should have a subject, verb, criteria for measurement, and a time when the subject is to have achieved the goal.

2. Applying a cotherapeutic, collaborative, client-centered view of the dental hygiene process of care, list strategies that can be utilized to involve and motivate the adolescent client in the care planning process.

REFERENCES

Academy for Sports Dentistry: Mouthguards essential for today's female athlete, 1999 (Online) *http://www.ada.org/public/media/newsrel/9910/nr-13.html* (accessed April 9, 2002).

Casamassimo PS, Griffiths P, Nowak A: Anticipatory guidance in dentistry. *Dental Hygienist News,* (5)2, 19–21, 1989.

Darby ML, Walsh MM: *Dental Hygiene Theory and Practice*, Philadelphia: Saunders, 1994, pp. 248–249, 343, 354–357.

Davis JR, Stegeman CA: *The Dental Hygienist's Guide to Nutritional Care.* Philadelphia: Saunders, 1998, pp. 363–378.

Debiase CB: *Dental Health Education: Theory and Practice.* Philadelphia: Lea & Febiger, 1991, pp. 105–121.

Fried JL: *The Dental Hygienist's Role in Tobacco Use, Prevention, and Cessation.* Chicago: American Dental Hygenists' Association Self Study Course, 1995.

Gulch-Scranton JZ, Tedisco AM: Individualizing dental hygiene patient management through out the life span. *Seminars in Dental Hygiene*. Yardley, PA: Professional Audience Communications, 1994.

Haring JI, Jansen L: *Dental Radiography Principles and Techniques*. Philadelphia: Saunders, 2000, pp. 370–373.

Hofman A, Glendanus D: *Adolescent Medicine*. Norwalk, CT: Appleton and Lange, 1989, pp. 21–32.

Horowitz HS, Driscoll WS, Meyers RJ, Heifetz SB, Kingman AK: A new method for assessing the prevalence of dental fluorosis. The tooth surface index of fluorosis. *Journal of the American Dental Association,* 109(7), 37, 1984.

Jacobson A, Caufield PW: *Introduction to Radiographic Cephalometry*. Philadelphia: Lea & Febiger, 1985, pp. 14–31.

Malamed SF: *Medical Emergencies in the Dental Office,* 5th ed. St. Louis: Mosby, 2000, pp. 36, 39–49, 214–221.

National Cancer Institute and National Institute of Dental Research: *Spitting into the Wind: The Facts about Dip and Chew.* Washington DC, U.S. Department of Health and Human Services, 1996.

Pinkham JR: *Pediatric Dentistry: Infancy Through Adolescence*. Philadelphia: Saunders, 1988, pp. 306–307, 342–343, 358-361, 455–456.

Slots J, Taubman M: *Contemporary Oral Microbiology and Immunology,* St. Louis: Mosby, 1993, p. 429.

Wilkins EM: *Clinical Practice of the Dental Hygienist,* 8th ed. Philadelphia: Lippincott Williams & Wilkins, 1999, pp. 110, 192, 254–261, 346–347, 455–479, 603–618, 677–678.

Woelful JB: *Dental Anatomy: Its Relevance to Dentistry,* 5th ed. Baltimore: Williams & Wilkins, 1997, pp. 100, 114.

Case C

Adult Periodontally Involved Client
Katherine Flynn

Learning Goals

Following integration of core scientific concepts and application of dental hygiene theory to the care of this client, the student will be able to

1. **Assess client characteristics.**
   A. Define classification of restorations.
   B. Identify the components of a removable partial denture.
   C. Recognize root caries risk factors.

2. **Obtain and interpret dental radiographs.**
   A. Determine dental materials type by their radiographic appearance.
   B. Identify radiographic artifacts.
   C. Distinguish normal radiographic anatomy and pathosis.
   D. Interpret periodontal pathology radiographically.

3. **Plan and manage dental hygiene care.**
   A. Prepare appropriately to prevent medical emergencies during treatment.
   B. Determine beneficial treatment interventions for the periodontally involved client.
   C. Recognize signs of anxiety regarding dental treatment.

4. **Perform periodontal procedures.**
   A. Determine periodontal risk factors that affect the severity and progression of periodontal disease.
   B. Determine clinical attachment levels (CAL).
   C. Identify mucogingival involvement risk factors.
   D. Identify disease sites that would be candidates for local drug delivery as adjunct therapies.
   E. Select appropriate drug delivery therapy.

5. **Use preventive agents.**
   A. Select appropriate adjunct therapies for hypersensitive root surfaces.
   B. Identify the rationale for fluoride therapies.

6. **Provide supportive treatment services.**
   A. Select appropriate pain control modality.
   B. Recommend appropriate therapy for parafunctional habits.

CLIENT'S HUMAN NEEDS DEFICITS

Because the client's oral wellness is interrelated with the client's attitudes toward health, values, and practices, and with family and cultural influences, it is important that the dental hygiene care plan be client-centered. Examination of human needs to assist the client in developing and maintaining appropriate self-care revealed the following deficits:

1. Protection from health risks

   Due to: Lack of oxygen to the brain

   Evidenced by: History of syncope and low blood pressure

2. Responsibility for oral health

   Due to: Arthritis pain

   Evidenced by: Client report

3. Skin and mucous membrane integrity of the head and neck

   Due to: Bacterial plaque and trauma from occlusion

   Evidenced by: Mucogingival involvement

4. Biologically sound dentition

   Due to: Decreased salivary production and root exposure

   Evidenced by: Dental caries and dentinal hypersensitivity

5. Freedom from anxiety and stress

   Due to: Apprehension regarding pain and embarrassment regarding fainting episodes

   Evidenced by: Rapid speech, nervous laughter, and overt enthusiasm

QUESTIONS

Basic Questions in Assessing Client Characteristics

1. Identify the classification of restoration for the maxillary left lateral incisor.
   A. Class I
   B. Class III
   C. Class IV
   D. Class V
   E. Class VI

Complex Questions in Assessing Client Characteristics

2. Which of the following abutment teeth support the removable partial denture rest?
   A. Maxillary first molars
   B. Maxillary anterior teeth
   C. Mandibular left second premolar and first molar
   D. Maxillary second premolars

3. All of the following are risk factors for this client's root caries EXCEPT one. Which one is the EXCEPTION?
   A. Prosthetic devices
   B. Medications
   C. Recession
   D. Bacterial plaque
   E. Fluoride history

Basic Questions in Obtaining and Interpreting Dental Radiographs

4. In addition to the composite restoration, which of the following dental materials is present on the maxillary right second premolar?
   A. Post and core
   B. Retention pins
   C. Silver points
   D. Gutta percha

5. The large radiopaque artifact present on the maxillary left lateral canine periapical radiograph and identified by the arrow is
   A. Cone cut error.
   B. Partial denture clasp.
   C. Amalgam tattoo.
   D. Film holding device.

6. Which of the following teeth presents with a composite restoration?
   A. Maxillary right first premolar
   B. Maxillary left first premolar
   C. Maxillary left second premolar
   D. Mandibular left first premolar
   E. Mandibular right second premolar

7. The round radiolucency visible near the apex of the mandibular left first premolar is MOST LIKELY
   A. Mental foramen.
   B. Residual cyst.
   C. Periapical abscess.
   D. Granuloma.

Complex Questions in Obtaining and Interpreting Dental Radiographs

8. The distal aspect of the mandibular right first molar reveals what periodontal condition?
   A. Periodontal abscess
   B. Vertical bone loss
   C. Furcation involvement
   D. Horizontal bone loss

Basic Questions in Planning and Managing Dental Hygiene Care

9. All of the following dental hygiene interventions will prevent the escalation of a medical emergency EXCEPT one. Which is the EXCEPTION?

    A. Resume upright chair position slowly after treatment.
    B. Set an ammonia capsule within easy reach during treatment.
    C. Provide prophylactic antibiotic premedication.
    D. Request client bring nitroglycerine to appointment.
    E. Develop good client rapport.

Complex Questions in Planning and Managing Dental Hygiene Care

10. Which of the following will increase success of non-surgical periodontal therapy for this client?

    A. Six-month recare interval
    B. Two half-mouth debridement appointments
    C. Instrumentation with universal curets
    D. Air-powder abrasive polishing

11. All of the following may be contributing to this client's dental anxiety EXCEPT one. Which is the EXCEPTION?

    A. Medications taken
    B. Past dental experiences
    C. Desire to appear in control
    D. Fear of pain
    E. Blood pressure

Basic Questions in Performing Periodontal Procedures

12. All of the following are periodontal risk factors for this client EXCEPT one. Which one is the EXCEPTION?

    A. Age
    B. Estrogen therapy
    C. Recession
    D. Tetracycline allergy
    E. Stress

13. The maxillary right canine has 4 mm of recession on the facial surface. What would be the clinical attachment loss for this tooth?

    A. 3 mm
    B. 4 mm
    C. 5 mm
    D. 6 mm
    E. 7 mm

14. Which of the following teeth are most at risk for mucogingival involvement?

    A. Maxillary right first premolar
    B. Maxillary right lateral incisor
    C. Maxillary left second premolar
    D. Mandibular left first molar
    E. Mandibular right lateral incisor

Complex Questions in Performing Periodontal Procedures

15. Based on the reassessment data from the 6-month recare appointment, which of the following teeth would be an ideal candidate for local drug delivery therapy?

    A. Maxillary right second molar
    B. Maxillary right first premolar
    C. Mandibular left first molar
    D. Mandibular left first premolar
    E. Mandibular right first molar

16. Which of the following local drug delivery agents would be most appropriate for this client?

    A. Minocycline capsule
    B. Doxycycline hyclate gel
    C. Chlorhexidine chip
    D. Doxycycline hyclate rinse

Complex Questions in Using Preventive Agents

17. Which of the following chemical agents would be MOST appropriate to recommend for at-home therapy to help alleviate the sensitivity of this client's teeth?

    A. Bonding agent
    B. Ferric oxylate
    C. Sodium fluoride
    D. Potassium nitrate
    E. Potassium oxylate

18. Which of the following is the overriding reason that this client should use home fluoride therapies?

    A. Bacterial plaque accumulations
    B. Salivary factors
    C. Frequency of sucrose in the diet
    D. Fluoride history

Basic Questions in Providing Supportive Treatment Services

19. Which of the following is the most appropriate form of pain control to be used during scaling and root debridement for this client?

    A. Topical benzocaine (Hurricane)
    B. Lidocaine transoral (Dentipatch)
    C. Injection lidocaine (Xylocaine)
    D. Oral diazepam (Valium)
    E. Nitrous oxide sedation

20. Due to the client's condition in the mandibular anterior region, which of the following would be the most effective supportive therapy to lessen tooth mobility?

    A. Fabrication of a nightguard
    B. Biofeedback to reduce parafunctional habits
    C. Therapeutic massage of tense muscles
    D. Splinting the teeth for stabilization

Answers appear on pages 77–80.

> ### *Reflective Activities*
>
> **1.** Describe methods of anxiety control that could be implemented for this client.
>
> **2.** Outline a plan of appointments addressing time needed, services planned, specific instruments, equipment necessary, and re-evaluation intervals for each appointment.
>
> **3.** Identify home care instructions to address the challenges associated with removable partial dentures, dentinal hypersensitivity, mucogingival involvement, and xerostomia.

REFERENCES

Blackwell RE: *G.V. Black's Operative Dentistry, Volume II,* 9th ed. Milwaukee: Medico-Dental Publishing, 1955, pp. 1–4.

Ciancio S: Local drug delivery of Chlorhexidine. *Compendium of Continuing Education in Dentistry,* 20(5), 427–431, 1999.

Darby ML, Walsh MM (eds): *Dental Hygiene Theory and Practice.* Philadelphia: Saunders, 1995, pp. 342–343.

Gage TW, Pickett FA: *Mosby's Dental Drug Reference,* 5th ed. St. Louis: Mosby, 2001, pp. 197–199, 209–210.

Genco RJ: Current view of risk factors for periodontal disease. *Journal of Periodontology,* 7, 1041–1049, 1996.

Hodges K: *Concepts in Nonsurgical Periodontal Therapy.* Albany, NY: Delmar, 1998, pp. 17, 58, 62, 97, 169, 319, 358–362.

Johnson L, Stoller N: Rationale for the use of Atridox® therapy for managing periodontal patients. *Compendium of Continuing Education in Dentistry,* 20(4) (Suppl.), 19–25, 1999.

Little JW, Falace DA, Miller, CS, Rhodus NL: *Dental Management of the Medically Compromised Patient.* St. Louis: Mosby, 1997, pp. 8–11, 197–202.

Malamed SF: *Medical Emergencies in the Dental Office,* 5th ed. St. Louis: Mosby, 2000, pp. 125–143.

Stamm JW, Banting DW, Imrey PB: Adult root caries survey of two similar communities with contrasting natural water levels. *Journal of the American Dental Association,* 120(2), 143–149, 1990.

Walker C: The supplemental use of antibiotics in periodontal therapy. *Compendium of Continuing Education in Dentistry,* 20(4) (Suppl.), 4–11, 1999.

Weinberg MA, Westphal C, Oakat M, Froum SJ: *Comprehensive Periodontology for the Dental Hygienist.* Upper Saddle River, NJ: Prentice Hall, 2001, pp. 176–178.

Wilkins EM: *Clinical Practice of the Dental Hygienist,* 8th ed. Philadelphia: Lippincott Williams & Wilkins, 1999, pp. 213, 232, 238, 241, 402, 736–760, 810–814.

Wilson TG, Glover ME, Schoen J, Baus C, Jacobs T: Compliance with maintenance therapy in a private periodontal practice. *Journal of Periodontology,* 55, 468–473, 1984.

Woodall IR: *Comprehensive Dental Hygiene Care,* 4th ed. St. Louis: Mosby, 1993, pp. 236–238.

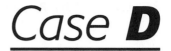

Case **D**

Adult Periodontally Involved Client
Louis Riddick

Learning Goals

Following integration of core scientific concepts and application of dental hygiene theory to the care of this client, the student will be able to

1. **Assess client characteristics.**
   A. Apply appropriate terminology to identify white lesions.
   B. Classify occlusal relationships.
   C. Identify deviations in gingival appearance.
   D. Determine etiology of diastema.

2. **Obtain and interpret dental radiographs.**
   A. Differentiate between normal radiographic anatomy and pathosis.
   B. Utilize radiographs as an aid in identifying periodontal disease risk factors.

3. **Plan and manage dental hygiene care.**
   A. Appropriately recommend a self-care product for the periodontally involved client.
   B. Individualize a treatment plan for the periodontally involved client.

4. **Perform periodontal procedures.**
   A. Recognize periodontal disease's effect on the dentition.
   B. Utilize periodontal instruments effectively.
   C. Describe bone loss patterns associated with periodontal disease.
   D. Classify furcation involvement according to severity.
   E. Measure clinical attachment level.
   F. Identify the predisposing factor in the presence of a periodontal pocket.
   G. Identify periodontal disease risk factors.
   H. Predict outcomes of periodontal disease treatment interventions.

5. **Use preventive agents.**
   A. Design appropriate professional smoking cessation follow-through services.

6. **Provide supportive treatment services.**
   A. Recommend appropriate recare interval for the periodontally involved client.

Situation

Louis Riddick and his wife owned and managed their own business until their sons took over last year. Now enjoying early retirement, Louis is still very active in his community. An easy-going, confident man, he has a close circle of friends with whom he enjoys playing golf. Recently diagnosed with mild hypertension, he is not overly concerned about his health. In fact, he has not had any dental care for several years. He is here today because his wife made the appointment for him after he mentioned that he thought his teeth might be getting loose.

For a detailed client history, including radiographs and color photos, see pages I-14 to I-17.

CLIENT'S HUMAN NEEDS DEFICITS

Because the client's oral wellness is interrelated with the client's attitudes toward health, values, and practices, and with family and cultural influences, it is important that the dental hygiene care plan be client-centered. Examination of human needs to assist the client in developing and maintaining appropriate self-care revealed the following deficits:

1. Protection from health risks

   Due to: Use of a prescribed smoking deterrent
   Evidenced by: Client self-report

2. Responsibility for oral health

   Due to: Lack of regular oral care
   Evidenced by: Periodontal disease and caries

   Due to: Neglecting the signs and symptoms of periodontal disease
   Evidenced by: Lack of awareness of the client's role in his own oral health

3. Skin and mucous membrane integrity of the head and neck

   Due to: Significant pocket depths
   Evidenced by: The presence of gingival inflammation and bleeding

4. Biologically sound dentition

   Due to: Potential for tooth loss
   Evidenced by: Tooth mobility

5. Conceptualization and understanding

   Due to: Misconceptions associated with oral health care
   Evidenced by: Lack of replacement of missing teeth

QUESTIONS

Basic Questions in Assessing Client Characteristics

1. Which of the following is the MOST LIKELY assessment of the soft tissue lesion located near the maxillary central incisors that does not wipe off with a gauze sponge?

A. Leukodema
B. Leukoplakia
C. Fordyce's granules
D. Nicotinic stomatitis
E. Candidiasis

2. Which of the following is the BEST assessment of this client's anterior occlusal relationship?

A. Underjet
B. Overjet
C. Crossbite
D. Edge-to-edge
E. Open bite

Complex Questions in Assessing Client Characteristics

3. The dark appearance of the facial gingiva is MOST LIKELY the result of

A. Melanin pigmentation.
B. Smoking stains.
C. Lichen planus.
D. Contact stomatitis.
E. Discoid lupus erythematosus.

4. Which of the following is the MOST LIKELY cause of this client's maxillary central diastema?

A. Enlarged incisive papilla
B. Periodontal involvement
C. Location of the frenal attachment
D. Tongue thrust
E. Developing radicular cyst

Basic Questions in Obtaining and Interpreting Dental Radiographs

5. Which of the following is the MOST LIKELY interpretation of the oval radiolucency between the maxillary central incisors?

A. Mental foramen
B. Mandibular foramen
C. Lingual foramen
D. Incisive foramen
E. Infraorbital foramen

Complex Questions in Obtaining and Interpreting Dental Radiographs

6. Which of the following is the MOST LIKELY interpretation of the radiopaque finding between the roots of the maxillary right first molar?

A. Composite restoration
B. Calculus
C. Hypercementosis
D. Enamel pearl
E. Pulp stone

Basic Questions in Planning and Managing Dental Hygiene Care

7. Which of the following would be the MOST beneficial oral self-care education for this client?

    A. Recommend modified Bass toothbrushing.
    B. Suggest using the dental floss holder.
    C. Introduce the end-tuft brush.
    D. Review skill enhancement with the automatic toothbrush.
    E. Provide a brochure on the interdental brush.

Complex Questions in Planning and Managing Dental Hygiene Care

8. Which of the following would MOST LIKELY be planned for this client's first appointment?

    A. Application of desensitizing agents
    B. Full-mouth periodontal scaling and root planing
    C. Extraction of the maxillary first molars
    D. Instruction in oral self-care
    E. Referral for evaluation of the white lesion

Basic Questions in Performing Periodontal Procedures

9. What factors contributed to the super eruption of the maxillary first molars?

    A. Furcation involvement
    B. Absence of mandibular first molars
    C. Long junctional epithelium
    D. Surgical intervention for periodontal disease
    E. Inadequate alveolar/attached gingiva

10. The purpose of the instrument shown in the photograph of the maxillary right first molar is to

    A. Measure furcation involvement.
    B. Scale posterior teeth.
    C. Explore for calculus.
    D. Record pocket depths.
    E. Apply subgingival irrigation.

11. Which of the following instruments would be the BEST choice for removing calculus on the mesial of the mandibular right second molar?

    A. Gracey 1/2 curet
    B. Gracey 11/12 curet
    C. Gracey 13/14 curet
    D. Universal sickle scaler
    E. Hirschfeld file

12. Which of the following BEST describes the type of bone loss associated with the maxillary right first and second premolars?

    A. Angular
    B. Vertical
    C. Horizontal
    D. Fenestration
    E. Dehiscence

13. Which of the following is the correct classification of furcation involving the maxillary right first molar?

    A. Grade I
    B. Grade II
    C. Grade III
    D. No furcation involvement present

14. What is the clinical attachment level present on the facial surface of the maxillary right first molar at the re-evaluation appointment?

    A. 10 mm
    B. 8 mm
    C. 6 mm
    D. 3 mm
    E. There is no loss of attachment present in this area.

Complex Questions in Performing Periodontal Procedures

15. Which of the following may be a contributing etiologic factor to the periodontal defect present on the mesial surface of the maxillary left first premolar?

    A. Endodontic therapy
    B. Overhanging amalgam restoration
    C. Incipient carious lesion
    D. Tooth root morphology
    E. Occlusal trauma

16. Which of the following is the MOST LIKELY cause of this client's tooth mobility?

    A. Periodontal disease
    B. Mild hypertension
    C. Chewing Nicorette®
    D. Premature loss of permanent teeth
    E. Smoking history

17. Which of the following has been the greatest risk factor for this client's periodontal disease?

    A. Brushing habits
    B. Medications
    C. Smoking
    D. Hypertension
    E. Stress

18. Which of the following is MOST LIKELY responsible for the reduction in pocket depths at the follow-up appointment?

    A. Tissue shrinkage
    B. Improved integrity of the clinical attachment
    C. Regeneration of the gingival tissue to normal color, size, and contour
    D. Long junctional epithelial attachment
    E. Connective tissue maturation

Complex Questions in Providing Supportive Treatment Services

19. Which of the following should be included in this client's smoking cessation follow-through from the dental hygienist?
    A. Provide positive reinforcement, emphasizing the benefits of stopping smoking.
    B. Warn the client that a single slip, smoking one cigarette, will make him a user again.
    C. Instruct him to chew nicotine gum as one would conventional chewing gum.
    D. Encourage limited use of nicotine gum throughout the day.
    E. Inform the client that nicotine withdrawal symptoms will subside in 5 to 7 days.

20. Based on the reassessment of this client, which of the following would be the BEST schedule for periodontal maintenance for this client?
    A. 1 month
    B. 3 months
    C. 6 months
    D. 9 months
    E. 12 months

Answers appear on pages 80–83.

Reflective Activities

1. Investigate tips and techniques to alleviate nicotine withdrawal symptoms that can be shared with clients.
2. Role play a script between the dental hygienist and a client who: (1) is not interested in quitting smoking; (2) thinks that switching from smoking cigarettes to using spit tobacco is beneficial; (3) is interested in quitting, but does not know how to begin.
3. Initiate a smoking cessation program (Ask, Advise, Assist, Arrange) with one of your clients who uses tobacco.

REFERENCES

Darby ML, Walsh MM (eds): *Dental Hygiene Theory and Practice*. Philadelphia: Saunders, 1995, pp. 956–957.

Glickman I: *Clinical Periodontology*. Philadelphia: Saunders, 1953.

Haber J, Kent RL: Cigarette smoking in a periodontal practice. *Journal of Periodontology*, 63(2), 100–106, 1992.

Hodges K: *Concepts in Nonsurgical Periodontal Therapy*. Albany, NY: Delmar, 1998, pp. 46–47.

National Institute of Health: *How to Help Your Patients Stop Using Tobacco*. National Cancer Society/National Cancer Institute, NIH Publication No. 93–3191, 1993.

Nield-Gehrig JS: *Fundamentals of Periodontal Instrumentation*, 4th ed. Baltimore: Lippincott Williams & Wilkins, 2000, pp. 205–210, 435–444.

Perry DA, Beemsterboer P, Taggart EJ: *Periodontology for the Dental Hygienist,* 2nd ed. Philadelphia: Saunders, 2001, pp. 130–131, 164–168, 228–229.

Weinberg MA, Westphal C, Palat M, Froum SJ: *Comprehensive Periodontics for the Dental Hygienist.* Upper Saddle River, NJ: Prentice Hall, 2001, pp. 379–395, 563–566.

Wilkins EM: *Clinical Practice of the Dental Hygienist,* 8th ed. Philadelphia: Lippincott Williams & Wilkins, 1999, pp. 425–438.

Learning Goals

Following integration of core scientific concepts and application of dental hygiene theory to the care of this client, the student will be able to

1. **Assess client characteristics.**
   A. Recognize etiology of deviations in gingival appearance.
   B. Distinguish normal anatomic features.
   C. Differentiate between caries, abrasion, and flexure lesions clinically.
   D. Determine the etiology of gingival recession.
   E. Identify risk factors for root caries.
   F. Be aware of oral manifestations of arthritis.

2. **Obtain and interpret dental radiographs.**
   A. Recognize dental materials radiographically.
   B. Apply appropriate radiographic technique corrective measures.
   C. Appropriately recommend the use of vertical or horizontal bitewing radiographs.
   D. Differentiate between normal radiographic anatomy and pathosis.

3. **Plan and manage dental hygiene care.**
   A. Identify prescribed medications and their effect on oral health.
   B. Modify oral healthcare treatment for the geriatric client.
   C. Select the appropriate dental hygiene procedure for treatment of the geriatric client.

4. **Perform periodontal procedures.**
   A. Classify periodontal status by type, location, and severity.
   B. Identify oral conditions that hinder instrumentation.
   C. Recommend appropriate follow-up care for the periodontally involved client.
   D. Plan scaling and root planing sequence.

5. **Use preventive agents.**
   A. Determine the need for appropriate supplemental oral hygiene devices and agents.

6. **Provide supportive treatment services.**
   A. Select the appropriate method for margination of an overhang amalgam.

Situation

Juan Hernandez enjoys coming to his regularly scheduled oral hygiene appointments. He is usually accompanied by his granddaughter, who drives him to his appointments. This client is ambulatory, with the use of a cane.

For a detailed client history, including radiographs and color photos, see pages I-18 to I-21.

CLIENT'S HUMAN NEEDS DEFICITS

Because the client's oral wellness is interrelated with the client's attitudes toward health, values, and practices, and with family and cultural influences, it is important that the dental hygiene care plan be client-centered. Examination of human needs to assist the client in developing and maintaining appropriate self-care revealed the following deficits:

1. Protection from health risks

   Due to: High blood pressure maintenance drugs
   Evidenced by: Client self-report

2. Biologically sound and functional dentition

   Due to: Future caries risk
   Evidenced by: Caries and xerostomia

3. Skin and mucous membrane integrity of the head and neck

   Due to: Presence of plaque
   Evidenced by: Bleeding on probing and periodontal disease

4. Responsibility for oral health

   Due to: Lack of daily home care
   Evidenced by: Periodontal disease and caries

5. Conceptualization and understanding

   Due to: Lack of awareness of need for more frequent brushing and interproximal removal of plaque
   Evidenced by: Client self-report brushing once a day and not flossing

QUESTIONS

Basic Questions in Assessing Client Characteristics

1. Which of the following best describes the bluish-colored gingival tissue lingual to the maxillary right first molar?
   A. Necrosis
   B. Cyanosis
   C. Leukoplakia
   D. Amalgam tattoo
   E. Exostosis

2. Which of the following is the MOST LIKELY assessment of this client's palate?

   A. Granular tumor
   B. Pseudocyst
   C. Gingival fibromatosis
   D. Torus palantinus
   E. Hyperplastic salivary ducts

Complex Questions in Assessing of Client Characteristics

3. In evaluating the buccal surfaces of the mandibular left canine, first premolar and second premolar areas, what would BEST describe the reason for the Class V restorations?

   A. Smooth surfaces caries
   B. Root caries
   C. Class I caries
   D. Toothbrush abrasion
   E. Abfraction lesions

4. Age and occlusal trauma are the cause of this client's gingival recession. This client's gingival recession has increased his risk of root caries.

   A. The first statement is true, and the second statement false.
   B. The first statement is false, and the second statement is true.
   C. Both statements are true.
   D. Both statements are false.

5. Which of the following may be a contributing factor in this client's temporomandibular joint (TMJ) dysfunction?

   A. History of a stroke
   B. High blood pressure
   C. Osteoarthritis
   D. Age
   E. Attrition

Basic Questions in Obtaining and Interpreting Dental Radiographs

6. The maxillary left second premolar shows signs of

   A. Endodontic therapy.
   B. Endosseous implant.
   C. Internal root resorption.
   D. Pulp stones.
   E. Apicoectomy.

7. Which one of the following would correct the technique error evidenced on the maxillary right canine periapical radiograph?

   A. Move the film posteriorly.
   B. Move the film anteriorly.
   C. Decrease the vertical angulation.
   D. Increase the vertical angulation.
   E. Move the PID inferiorly.

Complex Questions in Obtaining and Interpreting Dental Radiographs

8. Which of the following is the BEST reason for exposing vertical and not horizontal bitewing radiographs on this client?
   A. Advanced periodontal status
   B. Client's age
   C. Large tori present
   D. Temporomandibular disorder (TMD) limits opening
   E. Eliminates the need for periapical radiographs

9. Which of the following is the MOST LIKELY interpretation of the radiolucency observed near the mandibular right lateral incisor?
   A. Genial tubercles
   B. Mental foramen
   C. Periapical abscess
   D. Film identification dot
   E. Mandibular torus

Basic Questions in Planning and Managing Dental Hygiene Care

10. Which medication currently taken by this client may contraindicate proceeding with treatment today?
    A. Aspirin
    B. Coumadin
    C. Diuril
    D. Lipitor
    D. Naproxsyn

11. Which of the following would be contraindicated for this client?
    A. Periodontal therapies
    B. Air-powder abrasive polishing
    C. Ultrasonic instrumentation
    D. Nitrous oxide sedation
    E. Sodium fluoride application

Complex Questions in Planning and Managing Dental Hygiene Care

12. All of the following would provide effective communication with this client EXCEPT one. Which is the EXCEPTION?
    A. Remove face mask and face the client when speaking.
    B. Give frequent and immediate feedback regarding demonstration of home care techniques.
    C. Use simple drawings to explain dental procedures.
    D. When changing positions, move slowly around this client.
    E. Allow the client to get himself into position for treatment; provide assistance only when asked.

13. All of the following are important when planning oral health care appointments for this client EXCEPT one. Which is the EXCEPTION?
    A. Short appointments
    B. Frequent position changes
    C. Comfortable chair
    D. Physical supports such as pillows
    E. Morning appointments

14. All of the following may be recommended for this client EXCEPT one. Which is the EXCEPTION?

    A. Soft diet
    B. Moist heat to face/jaw
    C. Physician referral
    D. Occlusal appliance

Basic Questions in Performing Periodontal Procedures

15. Which of the following BEST describes this client's periodontal status?

    A. Gingivitis
    B. Localized moderate periodontitis
    C. Generalized moderate periodontitis
    D. Localized severe periodontitis
    E. Generalized severe periodontitis

16. All of the following may hinder scaling and root planing this client EXCEPT one. Which is the EXCEPTION?

    A. Furcation involvement
    B. Poorly contoured crown margins
    C. Cervical restorations
    D. Increased bleeding
    E. Cultural attitude

Complex Questions in Performing Periodontal Procedures

17. Based on this client's probing depths 1 month after scaling and root planing, all of the following would be indicated EXCEPT one. Which is the EXCEPTION?

    A. Perform periodontal surgery.
    B. Apply antibiotic therapy.
    C. Schedule a 6-month recare appointment.
    D. Instrument pockets and bleeding areas.
    E. Refer to a periodontist.

18. Which of the following would be the MOST appropriate treatment plan for this client?

    A. Four one-quadrant scaling and root planing appointments
    B. One half-mouth scaling and root planing per visit
    C. Complete mouth debridement, followed up with a complete mouth scaling and root planing appointment
    D. Gross scaling followed up with quadrant scaling and root planning appointments

Basic Questions in Using Preventive Agents

19. All of the following would be appropriate recommendations for this client's oral self-care program EXCEPT one. Which is the EXCEPTION?

    A. Automatic toothbrush
    B. Interproximal brushes
    C. Home fluoride rinse
    D. Oral irrigation device
    E. Floss holder

Basic Questions in Providing Supportive Treatment Services

20. Which of the following is the most effective procedure to improve the restoration present on the mesial of the maxillary right first molar?
    A. Smoothing using fine diamond interproximal finishing strips
    B. Removing using a flame-shaped silicon carbide bur
    C. Cutting by inserting a gold knife
    D. Trimming using a fine fluted pointed tungsten carbide bur

Answers appear on pages 83–86.

Reflective Activities

1. List 10 physiologic age-related changes of the human body and discuss their impact on dental hygiene treatment.

2. To simulate decreased manual dexterity, often encountered in the client with osteoarthritis, brush your teeth using your nondominant hand. (If you are right-handed, brush your teeth with your left hand.) Disclose and evaluate your plaque removal ability. Write an essay on how you would assist a client with reduced manual dexterity to perform oral home care.

3. List a belief about healthcare from your own cultural background. How does this belief assist in helping and/or hindering access to healthcare for the people of your culture?

REFERENCES

Alvarez KH: *Williams & Wilkins' Dental Hygiene Handbook.* Baltimore: Williams & Wilkins, 1998, pp. 326–333, 375–389.

Darby ML, Walsh MM (eds.): *Dental Hygiene Theory and Practice.* Philadelphia: Saunders, 1995, pp. 317, 553, 873–912.

Gage TW, Pickett FA: *Dental Drug Reference,* 5th ed. St. Louis: Mosby, 2001, pp. 55–56, 58, 135–136, 464–465, 712–713.

Little JW, Falce DA, Miller CS, Rhodus NL: *Dental Management of the Medically Compromised Patient,* 5th ed. St. Louis: Mosby, 1997, pp. 6–7, 28–31, 176–191, 363–366, 380–386.

Requa-Clark B: *Applied Pharmacology for the Dental Hygienist,* 4th ed. St. Louis: Mosby, 2000, pp. 321–364.

Wilkins EM: *Clinical Practice of the Dental Hygienist,* 8th ed. Philadelphia: Lippincott Williams & Wilkins, 1999, pp. 231–247, 634–645.

Learning Goals

Following integration of core scientific concepts and application of dental hygiene theory to the care of this client, the student will be able to

1. **Assess client characteristics.**
   A. Identify types of periodontal pockets.
   B. Classify case types of periodontal disease.
   C. Classify furcation involvement.
   D. Determine preliminary diagnosis of oral conditions that deviate from normal.

2. **Obtain and interpret dental radiographs.**
   A. Differentiate between a variety of normal radiographic anatomical landmarks.
   B. Interpret radiolucencies and radiopacities observed on a periapical radiograph.

3. **Plan and manage dental hygiene care.**
   A. Plan appropriate denture care based on the client's individualized needs.
   B. Recognize medical conditions that require antibiotic premedication.
   C. Identify appointment-planning considerations for the geriatric client.
   D. Identify effects of prescribed medications on oral and general health.
   E. Select appropriate interdental devices based on client needs.
   F. Select appropriate dental hygiene interventions based on individual needs.

4. **Perform periodontal procedures.**
   A. Differentiate between the severity of periodontal conditions that affect prognosis.
   B. Identify periodontal risk factors.
   C. Select appropriate scaling instruments for effective and efficient calculus removal.
   D. Recognize possible adverse effects of periodontal debridement.
   E. Predict treatment responses for the periodontally involved client.

5. **Use preventive agents.**
   A. Select treatment recommendations following reevaluation of initial periodontal debridement.

6. **Provide supportive treatment services.**
   B. Differentiate between acrylic products used in dental appliances.

> ### *Situation*
>
> Virginia Carson appears to struggle into the operatory and to get situated in the dental chair. She wheezes and appears out of breath with each movement. It has taken a lot of effort for her to get to the appointment today because she does not drive. She relies on the community's senior citizen transportation assistance to bring her to the dental office. The client knows that this appointment is necessary, but does not like "going to the dentist."
>
> *For a detailed client history, including radiographs and color photos, see pages I-22 to I-23.*

CLIENT'S HUMAN NEEDS DEFICITS

Because the client's oral wellness is interrelated with the client's attitudes toward health, values, and practices, and with family and cultural influences, it is important that the dental hygiene care plan be client-centered. Examination of human needs to assist the client in developing and maintaining appropriate self-care revealed the following deficits:

1. Protection from health risks

   Due to: Tobacco usage
   Evidenced by: Red and pin-pointed spots on palate

2. Responsibility for oral health

   Due to: Irregular dental visits
   Evidenced by: Heavy calculus deposits

3. Skin and mucous membrane integrity of the head and neck

   Due to: Bacterial plaque and inadequate oral health behaviors
   Evidenced by: The presence of gingival inflammation, pockets, and bleeding

   Due to: Chronic infection
   Evidenced by: Generalized redness of hard palate mucosa

4. Freedom from anxiety or stress

   Due to: Uneasiness regarding dental hygiene appointments
   Evidenced by: Client self-report

QUESTIONS

Basic Questions in Assessing Client Characteristics

1. Which of the following BEST describes the type of periodontal pocketing found on the mesial aspect of the mandibular left second premolar?
   A. Gingival pocket
   B. Pseudopocket
   C. Mucogingival pocket
   D. Infrabony pocket
   E. Suprabony pocket

2. Which of the following is the correct American Academy of Periodontology case type for this client?

   A. Class I
   B. Class II
   C. Class III
   D. Class IV
   E. Class V

Complex Questions in Assessing Client Characteristics

3. Identify the classification of furcation involvement of the mandibular right first molar.

   A. Grade I
   C. Grade II
   D. Grade III
   E. Grade IV
   F. Grade V

4. Which of the following is the MOST LIKELY assessment of the condition seen on this client's palate?

   A. Torus palatinus
   B. Melanin pigmentation
   C. Chronic atrophic candidiasis
   D. Primary herpetic gingivostomatitis
   E. Herpetiform apthous ulcers

Basic Questions in Obtaining and Interpreting Dental Radiographs

5. Which of the following describes the radiopaque circle, identified by the arrow, seen on the mandibular central incisor periapical radiograph?

   A. Retrocuspid papilla
   B. Symphysis
   C. Mental foramen
   D. Genial tubercles
   E. Trabeculae

6. What is the scalloped radiopaque line visible radiographically across the mandibular central incisors?

   A. Cementoenamel junction
   B. Calculus deposits
   C. Dense enamel layer
   D. Composite resin
   E. Cementicles

Complex Questions in Obtaining and Interpreting Dental Radiographs

7. Which of the following is the MOST LIKELY reason for the radiopaque appearance of the nasal fossa?

   A. Sinus infection
   B. Conchae present
   C. Film fog artifact
   D. Deviated septum
   E. Soft tissue of the nose imaged

8. Which one of the following is the MOST LIKELY interpretation of the radiolucency observed on the distal of the mandibular right first premolar?

   A. Caries
   B. Toothbrush abrasion
   C. Abfraction lesion
   D. Cervical burnout
   E. Root fracture

Basic Questions in Planning and Managing Dental Hygiene Care

9. Which of the following medical conditions predisposes this client for the need to premedicate with prophylactic antibiotic coverage?

   A. Bronchitis
   B. Hepatitis C
   C. Congestive heart failure
   D. Spontaneous gingival bleeding
   E. None of the above

10. To prevent stain accumulation on the client's new denture, which of the following home care regimens should the clinician recommend?

    A. Soak daily in an OTC mouthwash.
    B. Brush with a denture dentifrice using a denture brush.
    C. Immerse in full strength sodium hypochlorite overnight.
    D. Brush once a month using a household scouring powder.
    E. Clean with dishwasher detergent once every 6 months.

11. All of the following are appointment-planning considerations for this client EXCEPT one. Which is the EXCEPTION?

    A. Repeat self-care instructions.
    B. Select large-handled oral aids.
    C. Eliminate distracting music.
    D. Seat client in supine position.
    E. Face the client and speak clearly.

Complex Questions in Planning and Managing Dental Hygiene Care

12. All of the following are essential when planning oral health care appointments for this client EXCEPT one. Which is the EXCEPTION?

    A. Monitor vital signs.
    B. Avoid orthostatic hypotension.
    C. Assess salivary flow.
    D. Follow a stress reduction protocol.
    E. Use anesthesia with vasoconstrictor.

13. All of the following interdental devices would be beneficial for this client EXCEPT one. Which one is the LEAST BENEFICIAL?

    A. Saline irrigation
    B. Tufted dental floss
    C. Interdental tip
    D. Wooden interdental cleaner
    E. Toothpick in holder

14. Which one of the following interventions is MOST appropriate for this client?
    A. Tobacco cessation
    B. Oral cancer referral
    C. Dental implant evaluation
    D. Dietary counseling
    E. Advanced infection control procedures

Basic Questions in Performing Periodontal Procedures

15. Which of the following teeth presents with the poorest prognosis?
    A. Mandibular right second molar
    B. Mandibular right first premolar
    C. Mandibular right central incisor
    D. Mandibular left lateral incisor
    E. Mandibular left second premolar

16. Which one of the following instruments is the best choice for the removal of supragingival calculus from the lingual surfaces of this client's mandibular anterior teeth?
    A. Modified ultrasonic tip (slim design)
    B. Universal ultrasonic tip
    C. Universal curette scaler
    D. Area-specific root scaler
    E. Anterior sickle scaler

17. All of the following can be expected to delay healing following scaling EXCEPT one. Which is the EXCEPTION?
    A. Hepatitis C
    B. Medications
    C. Papillary shape
    D. Cigarette smoking
    E. Age

Complex Questions in Performing Periodontal Procedures

18. All of the following are increased possible adverse effects following periodontal debridement in this client EXCEPT one. Which is the EXCEPTION?
    A. Periodontal pockets
    B. Root caries
    C. Tooth mobility
    D. Dentinal hypersensitivity

Complex Questions in Using Preventive Agents

19. What additional therapy is MOST LIKELY to be recommended after evaluation of initial therapy?
    A. Surgical intervention
    B. Continued initial therapy
    C. Periodontal maintenance
    D. Restorative procedures
    E. Pit and fissure sealants

Basic Questions in Providing Supportive Treatment

20. Considering the clinical appearance of the maxillary denture, which of the following best describes the dental material used to manufacture it?
    A. Bis-phenol A-glycidal methacrylate (bis-GMA)
    B. Urethane dimethacrylate (UEDMA)
    C. Hydroxyethyl methacrylate (HEMA)
    D. Poly methyl methacrylate resin (MMA)
    E. Dipentaerythiol penta-acrylate monophosphate (PENTA-P)

Answers appear on pages 86–88.

Reflective Activities

1. Establish priorities in the dental and dental hygiene care plan. List factors that will influence the establishment of the dental hygiene care priorities (i.e., attitude of the client toward dental procedures, physical abilities, philosophy of the healthcare provider).

2. Discuss the client's multiple oral health maintenance needs and design a tailored self-care plan of devices and procedures that could be presented.

3. Design a stress reduction protocol that could be implemented for this client and others who require such attention.

REFERENCES

Anusavice KJ (ed.): *Phillips' Science of Dental Materials,* 10th ed. Philadelphia: Saunders, 1996, pp. 211–235.

Fried JL: *The Dental Hygienist's Role in Tobacco Use, Prevention and Cessation.* Chicago: ADHA Self Study Course, 1995.

Frommer HF: *Radiology for Dental Auxiliaries,* 7th ed. St. Louis: Mosby, 2001, pp. 312–365.

Gage TW, Pickett, FA. *Mosby's Dental Drug Reference,* 5th ed. St. Louis: Mosby, 2001, pp. 207–208, 232–234, 296–297.

Glickman I: *Clinical Periodontology.* Philadelphia: Saunders, 1953.

Haring JI, Jansen L: *Dental Radiography Principles and Techniques,* 2nd ed. Philadelphia: Saunders, 2000, pp. 411–439.

Hodges K: *Concepts in Nonsurgical Periodontal Therapy.* Boston: Delmar, 1997, pp. 289–344.

Ibsen OAC, Phelan JA: *Oral Pathology for the Dental Hygienist,* 3rd ed. Philadelphia: Saunders, 2000, pp. 103–176.

Little JW, Falce DA, Miller CS, Rhodus NL: *Dental Management of the Medically Compromised Patient,* 5th ed. St. Louis: Mosby, 1997, pp. 10–15, 231–240.

Perry DA, Beemsterboer P, Taggart EJ: *Periodontology for the Dental Hygienist,* 2nd ed. Philadelphia: Saunders, 2001, pp. 107–130.

Weinberg, MA, Westphal C, Pilat M, Froum SJ: *Comprehensive Periodontics for the Dental Hygienist.* Upper Saddle River, NJ: Prentice Hall, 2001, pp. 97, 133, 223–225, 238–257, 379–395, 608.

Wilkins EM: *Clinical Practice of the Dental Hygienist.* Philadelphia: Lippincott Williams & Wilkins, 1999, pp. 102, 230, 346–347, 370–393, 404–405, 432–435, 634–645, 795.

Case **G**

Special Needs Client
Thoroughgood Epps

Learning Goals

Following integration of core scientific concepts and application of dental hygiene theory to the care of this client, the student will be able to

1. **Assess client characteristics.**
   A. Identify dental materials.
   B. Determine possible oral side effects of medications.
   C. Classify restorations.
   D. Recognize dental restorative materials used to manufacture a dental prosthesis.

2. **Obtain and interpret dental radiographs.**
   A. Interpret findings on a dental radiograph.
   B. Evaluate data to assess dental materials and prostheses radiographically.

3. **Plan and manage dental hygiene care.**
   A. Apply appropriate dental hygiene treatment alterations for the client with degenerative joint disease.
   B. Select a dental hygiene care plan for scaling and root debridement.
   C. Incorporate appropriate self-care devices into preventive education disease management for the client with dental implants and fixed bridges.

4. **Perform periodontal procedures.**
   A. Determine periodontal maintenance intervals for the dental implant client.
   B. Identify the effect of untreated caries on periodontal tissue healing.
   C. Select appropriate assessment parameters for evaluating dental implants.
   D. Select dental hygiene instruments based on the client's assessment data.
   E. Determine appropriate hand instruments for periodontal debridement.

5. **Use preventive agents.**
   A. Select appropriate preventive agents based on client assessment data.
   B. Identify contraindications for using preventative agents/procedures given client characteristics.

6. **Provide supportive treatment services.**
   A. Recognize model trimming errors.
   B. Differentiate between different gypsum product formulations used for model fabrication.

Situation
Thoroughgood Epps is a neat, attractive, retired military officer. He is currently attending college to train for a new career since leaving the army. He is still being treated at a local Veteran's Hospital for osteoarthritis and became a dental implant candidate after a car accident three years ago.
For a detailed client history, including radiographs and color photos, see pages I-24 to I-27.

CLIENT'S HUMAN NEEDS DEFICITS

Because the client's oral wellness is interrelated with the client's attitudes toward health, values, and practices, and with family and cultural influences, it is important that the dental hygiene care plan be client-centered. Examination of human needs to assist the client in developing and maintaining appropriate self-care revealed the following deficits:

1. Protection from health hisks

    Due to: Risk for aggravating osteoarthritis

    Evidenced by: Previous neck injury

    Due to: Risk for prolonged hemorrhage

    Evidenced by: Use of nonsteroidal antinflammatory drugs (NSAIDs) to control arthritis inflammation

2. Responsibility for oral health

    Due to: Lack of appropriate self-care

    Evidenced by: Generalized interproximal and subgingival plaque

    Due to: Neglecting the signs and symptoms of gingivitis

    Evidenced by: His focus on dental implant care and neglect of the remainder of his oral cavity

3. Skin and mucous membrane integrity of the head and neck

    Due to: Insufficient plaque removal

    Evidenced by: The presence of 4 to 5 mm pocket depths and localized moderate bleeding on probing

4. Biologically sound dentition

    Due to: Insufficient interproximal plaque removal

    Evidenced by: Proximal surface carious lesion

QUESTIONS

Basic Questions in Assessing Client Characteristics

1. The restorative treatment of the mandibular anterior teeth is best described as a(n)
    A. Removable partial denture.
    B. Gold bar and overdenture.
    C. Implant superstructure.

D. Periodontal splint.

E. Lingual retainer.

2. The restorative treatment of the maxillary left first molar is termed

A. Abutment.

B. Pontic.

C. Veneer.

D. Cantilever.

E. Crown.

3. What is the class of restoration that is observed on the mandibular left first molar?

A. Class I

B. Class II

C. Class III

D. Class IV

E. Class V

Complex Questions in Assessing Client Characteristics

4. The dental hygienist should examine this client for which of the following possible oral side effects of his medication?

A. Glossitis

B. Candidiasis

C. Gingival hyperplasia

D. Xerostomia

E. Black hairy tongue

5. Which of the following is the reason why the left side of the mandibular anterior restorative treatment does not appear to be attached to the adjacent natural tooth?

A. Implant failure

B. Resorption of the implant

C. Cantilever pontic

D. Temporary crown

E. Second premolar is periodontally involved

6. From which of the following dental materials were the client's implants manufactured?

A. Surgical steel screws

B. Chrome-cobalt framework

C. Plasma-sprayed titanium cylinders

D. Gold alloy pontics

E. Tungsten carbide blades

Complex Questions in Obtaining and Interpreting Dental Radiographs

7. Which of the following types of implants does this client present with?

A. Endosseous

B. Subperiosteal

C. Transosteal

D. Endodontic

E. Mandibular staple

8. Which of the following conditions is observed in the pulp chamber of the mandibular right first molar?

    A. Enamel pearl
    B. Secondary dentin
    C. Condensing osteitis
    D. Hypercementosis
    E. Abscess

Complex Questions in Planning and Managing Dental Hygiene Care

9. Which of the following treatment considerations is most appropriate for this client's medical conditions?

    A. Seat in semisupine position during treatment.
    B. Schedule appointment times in the morning.
    C. Use the immobile client transfer.
    D. Consult with his physician prior to scaling.
    E. Adjust chair to client's tolerance level.

10. Which of the following is the most appropriate dental hygiene care plan for this client's periodontal condition?

    A. One hour appointment of scaling to remove calculus and stain followed by a maintenance appointment in 6 months
    B. Two 1-hour appointments of gross scale at first appointment and fine scale at final appointment followed by a re-evaluation in 3 months
    C. Two 1-hour appointments for scaling and root debridement followed by a re-evaluation in 4 to 6 weeks
    D. Four 1-hour appointments for quadrant scaling and root debridement followed by a re-evaluation in 4 to 6 weeks

11. To improve plaque control, which one of the following oral hygiene devices would you recommend to replace the client's use of toothpicks?

    A. Wooden wedges
    B. Powered flossing device
    C. End-tuft brush
    D. Interproximal brush
    E. Tufted floss

Basic Questions in Performing Periodontal Procedures

12. Which of the following probes should be utilized in the mandibular anterior region for this client?

    A. Plastic probe
    B. Nabor's probe
    C. Goldman-Fox probe
    D. Michigan "O" probe

Complex Questions in Performing Periodontal Procedures

13. Which risk factor may have caused the lack of tissue response of the mesial of the mandibular left first molar area at the 4-week reevaluation appointment?

    A. Inappropriate time interval for tissue response
    B. Bacterial seeding from dental caries
    C. Past radiation exposure

D. Undetected systemic conditions

E. Xerostomia

14. What is the appropriate length of time between periodontal maintenance appointments for this client's recare?

A. 1 to 2 month intervals

B. 3 to 4 month intervals

C. 6-month intervals

D. Once a year

E. A personalized schedule

15. Which of the following is the MOST reliable indicator of this client's implant success?

A. Gingival color

B. Bleeding on probing

C. Pocket depths

D. Mobility

E. Papillary shape

16. Which of the following hand-activated instruments would be the best choice for debridement of the client's right posterior sextants?

A. Area-specific Gracey curet scalers

B. Universal curet scaler

C. Universal sickle scaler

D. Graphite curet scaler

E. Periodontal file

Complex Questions in Using Preventive Agents

17. Considering the oral findings, which of the following preventive agents will benefit this client the most?

A. Pit and fissure sealants

B. Stannous fluoride toothpaste

C. Chlorhexidine gluconate mouth rinse

D. Low-potency OTC fluoride rinse

E. Administration of potassium oxalate

18. Which of the following preventive procedures are contraindicated for this client?

A. Mouth rinses containing alcohol

B. Topical acidulated phosphate fluoride

C. Tartar control dentifrice

D. Application of disclosing solution

E. Intraoral radiographs

Basic Questions in Providing Supportive Treatment Services

19. Which of the following gypsum products was used to construct the client's diagnostic casts?

A. Calcium sulfate dihydrate

B. Calcium sulfate hemihydrate

C. Calcium sulfate alpha-hemihydrate

D. Calcium sulfate beta-hemihydrate

20. Which of the following trimming errors is evident on this client's diagnostic casts?
    - A. Tooth structure has been trimmed away.
    - B. Diagnostic cast is not parallel to the occlusal plane.
    - C. Lower right second molar is broken off the cast.
    - D. There is excess stone in the periphery.
    - E. Base is too thin on the right side of maxillary cast.

Answers appear on pages 89–91.

Reflective Activities

1. Describe the best implant instrument design, stroke direction, and amount of lateral pressure used for:
   - **a.** Debridement of the apical portion of the prosthetic framework.
   - **b.** Assessment of the periodontal tissues.
   - **c.** Debridement of the abutment posts.
   - **d.** Subgingival debridement.
2. Describe a plan for debridement that addresses this client's risk for prolonged bleeding. Specify armamentarium, time frames, sextants, medicinal agents, physician consultations, debridement instruments, etc.

REFERENCES

Anusavice KJ: Efficacy of non-surgical management of the initial caries lesion. *Journal of Dental Education,* 61, 895–905, 1997.

Anusavice KJ: *Phillips' Science of Dental Materials,* 10th ed. Philadelphia: Saunders, 1996, pp. 186–188, 657–662.

Blackwell RE: *GV Black's Operative Dentistry, Vol II,* 9th ed. Milwaukee: Medico Dental Publishing, 1955, pp. 1–4.

Daniels A: The importance of accurate charting for maintaining dental implants. *Practical Hygiene,* 2(5), 9–12, 1993.

Darby ML, Walsh MM: *Dental Hygiene Theory and Practice.* Philadelphia: Saunders, 1994, pp. 342–343, 359–360, 494–495, 642.

Gage TW, Pickett FA: *Mosby's Dental Drug Reference,* 5th ed. St Louis: Mosby, 2001, pp. 356–357.

Hodges KO: *Concepts in Nonsurgical Periodontal Therapy,* Albany, NY: Delmar, 1998, pp. 394–402.

Little JW, Falace DA, Miller CS, Rhodus NL: *Dental Management of the Medically Compromised Patient.* St. Louis: Mosby, 1992, p. 321.

Nield-Gehrig JS: *Fundamentals of Periodontal Instrumentation,* 4th ed. Philadelphia: Lippincott Williams & Wilkins, 2000, pp. 199–210, 531–536.

Perry DA, Beemsterboer PL, Taggart EJ: *Periodontology for the Dental Hygienist.* Philadelphia: Saunders, 1996, pp. 258–275.

Phinney DJ, Halstead JH: *Essential Skills and Procedures for Chairside Dental Assisting.* Albany, NY: Delmar, 2002, p. 55.

Twetman S, Peterson LG: Comparison of the efficacy of three different chlorhexidine preparations in decreasing the levels of *mutans streptococci* in saliva and interdental plaque. *Caries Research,* 32(2),113–118, 1998.

Weinberg MA, Westphal C, Palat M, Froum SJ: *Comprehensive Periodontics for the Dental Hygienist.* Upper Saddle River, NJ: Prentice Hall, 2001, pp. 513–537.

Wilkins EM: *Clinical Practice of the Dental Hygienist,* 8th ed. Philadelphia: Lippincott Williams & Wilkins, 1999, pp. 182, 237, 259, 421, 689, 785.

Woodall IR: *Comprehensive Dental Hygiene Care,* 4th ed. St. Louis: Mosby, 1993, pp. 236–238.

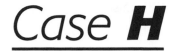

Case *H*

Special Needs Client
"Johnnie" Johnson

Learning Goals

Following integration of core scientific concepts and application of dental hygiene theory to the care of this client, the student will be able to

1. **Assess client characteristics.**
   A. Identify nicotine stomatitis.
   B. Distinguish anatomic characteristics of the periodontium.
   C. Identify the risk factors for oral cancer.
   D. Recognize oral conditions and characteristics resulting from excessive alcohol intake.
   E. Determine the effect of sialadenosis on the oral cavity.

2. **Obtain and interpret dental radiographs.**
   A. Interpret radiographic deviation from normal anatomic conditions.
   B. Identify suspected carious lesions radiographically.

3. **Plan and manage dental hygiene care.**
   A. Provide the appropriate preprocedural rinse for the alcoholic client.
   B. Counsel the vitamin deficient client for sources of folic acid.
   C. Recognize the etiology of multiple carious lesions.
   D. Plan treatment for the client with multiple caries.
   E. Make ethical decisions when treating the alcoholic dental client.
   F. Appropriately manage professional oral healthcare treatment for the special needs client.
   G. Identify barriers to professional oral healthcare treatment.
   H. Identify contraindications for administration of professional oral healthcare treatment.

4. **Perform periodontal procedures.**
   A. Apply standard and advanced fulcruming techniques.
   B. Sequence periodontal intervention procedures.

5. **Provide supportive treatment services.**
   A. Recommend appropriate behaviors that will lead to improved health.
   B. Refer the special needs client for the appropriate supportive treatment.

Situation

"Johnnie" Johnson works as a disk jockey in dance clubs and for hire at other functions and parties. He admits to heavy drinking and "a lot of partying." His alcohol consumption appears to be affecting his physical appearance. His hands tremor slightly and he speaks rapidly and nervously. He does not appear to be intoxicated at this time; however, his breath indicates recent alcohol consumption.

For a detailed client history, including radiographs and color photos, see pages I-28 to I-29.

CLIENT'S HUMAN NEED DEFICITS

Because the client's oral wellness is interrelated with the client's attitudes toward health, values, and practices, and with family and cultural influences, it is important that the dental hygiene care plan be client-centered. Examination of human needs to assist the client in developing and maintaining appropriate self-care revealed the following deficits:

1. Protection from health risks

   Due to: Alcoholism
   Evidenced by: Appearance, tremors, and breath

2. Biologically sound and functional dentition

   Due to: Neglect of professional oral care
   Evidenced by: Multiple dental caries and defective restorations

3. Skin and mucous membrane integrity of the head and neck

   Due to: Xerostomia and gingival bleeding upon probing
   Evidenced by: Parotid gland enlargement

4. Freedom from anxiety or stress

   Due to: Financial burden of dental treatment
   Evidenced by: Cancelled or broken appointments

5. Responsibility for oral health

   Due to: Inadequate professional oral health care
   Evidenced by: No dental exam within the past 10 to 15 years

QUESTIONS

Basic Questions in Assessing Client Characteristics

1. The client's palate has diffuse small, red dots which are indicative of
   A. Nicotine stomatitis.
   B. Hyperkeratosis.
   C. Pyogenic granuloma.
   D. Kaposi's sarcoma.
   E. Trauma from hot food.

2. The deeper red tissue on the facial aspect of the mandibular anterior region is called
   A. Free gingiva.
   B. Attached gingiva.
   C. Oral epithelium.
   D. Junctional epithelium.
   E. Alveolar mucosa.

Complex Questions in Assessing Client Characteristics

3. Which of the following contributes to this client's increased risk for oral carcinoma?
   A. Use of multiple antacids
   B. High pulse and respiration rate
   C. Xerostomia conditions
   D. Alcohol use and smoking
   E. Rampant caries with abscesses

4. This client exhibits all of the following that may indicate alcohol withdrawal syndrome EXCEPT one. Which is the EXCEPTION?
   A. Hand tremors
   B. Rapid pulse
   C. Xerostomia
   D. Craving antacids
   E. Swollen glands

5. Painless, benign, bilateral parotid swellings frequently accompany chronic alcohol use. The reduced salivary output has allowed this client's dental caries to spread between adjacent teeth.
   A. The first statement is correct. The second statement is incorrect.
   B. The first statement is incorrect. The second statement is correct.
   C. Both statements are correct.
   D. Both statements are incorrect.

Complex Questions in Obtaining and Interpreting Radiographs

6. The radiolucency observed at the apex of the mandibular left lateral incisor is MOST LIKELY
   A. Periapical abscess.
   B. Condensing osteitis.
   C. Residual cyst.
   D. Lingual foramen.

7. All of the following teeth exhibit caries EXCEPT one. Which is the EXCEPTION?
   A. Maxillary right lateral incisor
   B. Maxillary right central incisor
   C. Maxillary left central incisor
   D. Mandibular left central incisor
   E. Mandibular left lateral incisor

Basic Questions in Planning and Managing Dental Hygiene Care

8. A nonalcohol preprocedural rinse is indicated due to this client's alcohol use pattern.

   A. Both the statement and reason are correct and related.
   B. Both the statement and reason are correct but not related.
   C. The statement is correct but the reason is not.
   D. The statement is not correct but the reason is accurate.
   E. Neither the statement nor reason is correct.

9. Which of the following can be added to this client's diet to address his vitamin deficiency?

   A. Folic acid supplements
   B. Liver and kidney organ meats
   C. Green vegetables
   D. Multiple vitamins
   E. Sunlight exposure

10. Based on this client's history and exam findings, which of the following is the best dental hygiene intervention?

    A. Tell him to take vitamin supplements.
    B. Recommend an Ensure® drink daily.
    C. Provide salivary substitutes.
    D. Advise him to eat more frequently.
    E. Counsel him for weight management.

Complex Questions in Planning and Managing Dental Hygiene Care

11. Although the client has arrived for his dental appointment smelling of alcohol, his speech is not slurred and his gait is steady. The dental hygienist has chosen to treat him for a quadrant scaling appointment. What is the basis for this decision?

    A. He has decision-making capacity.
    B. He has chosen to reveal his alcohol problem.
    C. The dental hygienist is covered by malpractice insurance.
    D. The dental hygienist is using the right of therapeutic privilege.
    E. This client should not be treated today.

12. Which of the following is the leading cause of this client's multiple carious lesions?

    A. Self-treatment of ulcers
    B. Xerostomia
    C. Accelerated pulse and respiration rate
    D. Tobacco use
    E. Poor oral hygiene

13. The client's oral condition requires interventions by the dental hygienist. Which of the following would best serve him?

    A. Fluoride supplementation
    B. Salivary substitutes and stimulants
    C. Tobacco cessation program
    D. Tooth-whitening procedures
    E. Nutritional counseling

14. Which of the following should be considered when treating this client?
    A. Chair positioning
    B. Alcohol withdrawal syndrome
    C. Spontaneous gingival bleeding
    D. Reducing microbial aerosols

15. Which of the following is the MOST LIKELY reason this client has difficulty keeping his scheduled dental hygiene appointments?
    A. Lack of knowledge regarding the importance of oral health
    B. Negative dental experience as a child
    C. Preoccupation with drinking
    D. Fear of being in pain

Basic Questions in Performing Periodontal Procedures

16. When scaling the maxillary left posterior buccal aspects, the clinician should refrain from fulcruming
    A. In the maxillary left canine/premolar area.
    B. With the palm of the hand on the client's chin.
    C. On the tooth adjacent to the area being instrumented.
    D. On the maxillary left incisors.

Complex Questions in Performing Periodontal Procedures

17. Following the phase of periodontal procedure sequencing where periapical emergencies are treated, this client will enter which of the following treatment phases?
    A. Preliminary phase
    B. Etiotropic phase
    C. Surgical phase
    D. Maintenance phase

Basic Questions in Providing Supportive Treatment Services

18. The client's teeth are in need of cosmetic dental restorative treatment. He would be a good candidate for tooth whitening.
    A. Both statements are TRUE.
    B. Both statements are FALSE.
    C. The first statement is TRUE. The second statement is FALSE.
    D. The first statement is FALSE. The second statement is TRUE.

Complex Questions in Providing Supportive Treatment Services

19. All of the following should be recommended for this client EXCEPT one. Which is the EXCEPTION?
    A. Reduce alcohol consumption.
    B. Reduce cigarette smoking.
    C. Increase nutritional balance.
    D. Increase frequency of dental hygiene care.
    E. Increase use of calcium carbonate.

20. Which of the following should be this client's FIRST referral?
    A. Endodontist
    B. Dietician
    C. Physician
    D. Alcoholism recovery group
    E. Smoking cessation classes

Answers appear on pages 92–95.

Reflective Activities

1. Alcoholic individuals have an increased rate of oral cancer. Plan a smoking cessation program for this client.

2. Alcoholism results in poor nutrition and folic acid deficiency. Assess this client's eating habits and plan incorporation of folic acid.

3. Role play how the clinician could approach this client about the importance of regular physical examinations.

4. In a small group activity, brainstorm all of the possible reasons for why this individual avoids dental care and then identify how the dental hygienist might address each of these.

REFERENCES

Alvarez K: *Dental Hygiene Handbook.* Baltimore: Williams and Wilkins, 1998, pp. 419–421.

Gage TW, Pickett FA: *Mosby's Dental Drug Reference,* 5th ed. St. Louis: Mosby, 2001, pp. 328–330.

Ibsen OAC, Phelan J: *Oral Pathology for the Dental Hygienist,* 3rd ed. Philadelphia: WB Saunders, 2000, pp. 64, 66, 75, 276.

Langlais RP, Miller CS: *Color Atlas of Common Oral Disease,* 2nd ed. Philadelphia: Williams and Wilkins, 1998, pp. 48–51, 72–73, 76, 86–87, 164.

Medical Economics: *Physicians Desk Reference for Nonprescription Drugs and Dietary Supplements,* 22nd ed. Montvale, NJ: Thomson Healthcare, 2001, pp. 636, 638, 673–674.

Miller RL, Gould AR, Bernstein ML, Read CJ: *General Pathology for the Dental Hygienist.* St. Louis: Mosby, 1995, pp. 200–201, 254–260.

Nizel A, Papas A: *Nutrition in Clinical Dentistry,* 3rd ed. Philadelphia: Saunders, 1989, p. 106.

Weinstein B: *Dental Ethics.* Philadelphia: Lea & Febiger, 1993, p. 69.

Wilkins E: *Clinical Practice of the Dental Hygienist,* 8th ed. Philadelphia: Lippincott Williams & Wilkins, 2000, pp. 836–845, 931.

Case **I**

Medically Compromised Client
Thomas Small

Learning Goals

Following integration of core scientific concepts and application of dental hygiene theory to the care of this client, the student will be able to

1. Assess client characteristics.
   A. Determine the etiology of gingival inflammation.
   B. Recognize factors which contribute to the creation of nonpathologic oral deviations from normal.
   C. Utilize standard indices in assessing periodontal health.
   D. Identify variants of normal head and neck anatomy.
   E. Determine the effects of medications on the oral cavity.

2. Obtain and interpret dental radiographs.
   A. Identify normal radiographic anatomy.
   B. Recognize radiographic artifacts.
   C. Recognize common anatomic anomalies observed in radiographs.

3. Plan and manage dental hygiene care.
   A. Prescribe an appropriate self-care method for the mildly retarded client.
   B. Plan optimal dental hygiene treatment for the client with seizure disorder.
   C. Select appropriate treatment regimens for the client with seizure disorder.
   D. Determine the ability of the client to give informed consent.

4. Perform periodontal procedures.
   A. Select the most appropriate calculus removal method.
   B. Identify the pathogenesis of periocoronitis.
   C. Select appropriate adjunctive therapy for periodontal disease as it relates to pericornitis.
   D. Evaluate the prognosis of oral health care instruction and scaling on the gingival condition.

5. Use preventive agents.
   A. Identify contraindications for the use of chemotherapeutics.

6. Provide supportive treatment services.
   A. Select the appropriate local anesthesia injection.
   B. Prepare for a medical emergency in response to an epileptic seizure.

> ### *Situation*
>
> Thomas Small always presents for his oral healthcare appointments with an eager seriousness. He likes to have all procedures explained in detail prior to consenting to treatment.
>
> *For a detailed client history, including radiographs and color photos, see pages I-30 to I-31.*

CLIENT'S HUMAN NEEDS DEFICITS

Because the client's oral wellness is interrelated with the client's attitudes toward health, values, and practices, and with family and cultural influences, it is important that the dental hygiene care plan be client-centered. Examination of human needs to assist the client in developing and maintaining appropriate self-care revealed the following deficits:

1. Protection from health risks

    Due to: High blood pressure
    Evidenced by: Use of multiple anticonvulsant drugs

    Due to: Potential for epileptic seizure from loud noise
    Evidenced by: Self-report regarding last seizure

2. Responsibility for oral health

    Due to: Inadequate toothbrushing
    Evidenced by: Lack of a toothbrush

3. Skin and mucous membrane integrity of the head and neck

    Due to: Gingival inflammation
    Evidenced by: Spontaneous bleeding

4. Conceptualization and understanding

    Due to: Mild mental retardation
    Evidenced by: Documented medical history and report of caregiver

QUESTIONS

Basic Questions in Assessing Client Characteristics

1. Which of the following BEST describes the enlarged gingiva in the anterior region?
    A. Phenytoin-related hyperplasia
    B. Hyperkeratinized gingiva
    C. Stillman's cleft
    D. Melanin pigmentation
    E. McCall's festooning

2. The appearance of the facial gingiva adjacent to the maxillary left lateral incisor and maxillary left canine indicate that the plaque accumulation has been in this area for
    A. Less than 24 hours.
    B. 1 to 5 days.

C. 5 to 10 days.

D. 10 to 15 days.

Complex Questions in Assessing Client Characteristics

3. According to the Plaque Index of Silness and Loe, which of the following scores would be applied to this client's maxillary anterior teeth?

   A. 0

   B. 1

   C. 2

   D. 3

4. All of the following may be contributing to this client's cheilosis EXCEPT one. Which is the EXCEPTION?

   A. Slight retardation

   B. Medications taken

   C. Seizure disorder

   D. Licking the lips

   E. Mouth breathing

5. Which of the following is the MOST LIKELY assessment of the nodule-like finding located on the facial gingiva, adjacent to the maxillary right second premolar?

   A. Papilloma

   B. Neuroma

   C. Exostosis

   D. Parulis

   E. Fibroma

Basic Questions in Obtaining and Interpreting Dental Radiographs

6. Which of the following is the MOST LIKELY interpretation of the long tubelike radiolucency observed in the mandibular right molar periapical radiograph?

   A. Compound fracture

   B. Nutrient canal

   C. Internal oblique ridge

   D. Mylohyoid line

   E. Mandibular canal

7. Which of the following radiographic artifacts is seen on the maxillary left molar periapical radiograph?

   A. Torn emulsion

   B. Static electricity

   C. Roller marks

   D. Fixer spill

   E. Fingernail marks

Complex Questions in Obtaining and Interpreting Dental Radiographs

8. Which of the following is the MOST LIKELY interpretation of the anomalies observed in the maxillary molar periapical radiographs?

   A. Bony exostosis

   B. Dens invaginatus

   C. Enamel pearl

   D. Supernumerary teeth

   E. Impacted third molars

Basic Questions in Planning and Managing Dental Hygiene Care

9. All of the following should be considered when treating this client, EXCEPT one. Which is the EXCEPTION?

   A. Include a mouth prop in the treatment armamentarium.
   B. Schedule appointments within the first few hours of daily medications.
   C. Ask the client to report aura sensation immediately upon sensing.
   D. Ready life support oxygen for respiratory support.
   E. Prepare to administer cardiopulmonary resuscitation (CPR).

10. Which of the following treatment regimens is contraindicated for this client?

    A. Coronal polishing
    B. Subgingival irrigation
    C. Ultrasonic scaling
    D. Root planing
    E. Toothbrush deplaquing

Complex Questions in Planning and Managing Dental Hygiene Care

11. Which of the following oral home care recommendations would be MOST LIKELY to motivate this client to improve his oral self-care technique?

    A. Disclose and show plaque accumulation using a hand mirror.
    B. Provide a brochure with large pictures demonstrating brushing technique.
    C. Give him a toothbrush with his name on it.
    D. Include the group home supervisor in oral self-care instructions.
    E. Utilize a digital intraoral camera that images the oral cavity on a monitor.

12. Which of the following should be performed prior to subgingival scaling?

    A. Premedicate with appropriate antibiotics.
    B. Determine pretreatment bleeding time.
    C. Prescribe nonsteroidal antiinflammatory drugs (NSAIDs).
    D. Rinse with an alcohol containing mouth rinse.
    E. Irrigate subgingivally with saline.

13. This client is able to give informed consent for oral surgery to remove the impacted teeth BECAUSE he has decision-making capacity.

    A. Both the statement and reason are correct and related.
    B. Both the statement and reason are correct but not related.
    C. The statement is correct but the reason is not.
    D. The statement is not correct but the reason is accurate.
    E. Neither the statement nor reason is correct.

Basic Questions in Performing Periodontal Procedures

14. All of the following microorganisms are associated with this client's odontogenic infection EXCEPT one. Which is the EXCEPTION?

    A. Bacteroides
    B. Fusobacterium
    C. *Streptococcus milleri*
    D. *Streptococcus mutans*
    E. *Peptostreptococcus*

15. Which of the following is indicated for the brown spot on the maxillary right first premolar?

    A. Subgingival irrigation with an antimicrobial agent
    B. Polishing with a medium-grit abrasive
    C. Toothbrushing with a fluoridated dentifrice
    D. Scaling with a universal curet

Complex Questions in Performing Periodontal Procedures

16. Which of the following treatment regimens is appropriate for this client's pericornitis at this appointment?

    A. Scaling debridement
    B. Doxycycline chemotherapy
    C. Extraction of impacted teeth
    D. Saline irrigation
    E. Antibiotic coverage

17. Following debridement and plaque control instructions, what reduction in probing depths can be expected at the 1 month evaluation appointment?

    A. 0 to 1 mm
    B. 2 to 3 mm
    C. 4 to 5 mm
    D. Increased probing depths

Complex Questions in Using Preventive Agents

18. This client's periodontal condition is influenced by the carbamazepine he takes for convulsions. Carbamazepine interacts with doxycycline and contraindicates its post-scaling use in his posterior periodontal pockets.

    A. Both statements are true.
    B. Both statements are false.
    C. The first statement is true. The second statement is false.
    D. The first statement is false. The second statement is true.

Basic Questions in Providing Supportive Treatment Services

19. All of the following should be executed if this client begins to exhibit uncontrolled muscle motor movements EXCEPT one. Which is the EXCEPTION?

    A. Monitor vital signs
    B. Provide aggressive restraints
    C. Place in a supine position
    D. Place client on his side
    E. Protect head from trauma

20. When scaling the maxillary right first premolar, which nerve should receive local anesthesia injection?

    A. Infraorbital
    B. Anterior superior alveolar
    C. Middle superior alveolar
    D. Posterior superior alveolar
    E. Greater palatine

Answers appear on pages 95–97.

Reflective Activities

1. Discuss a case situation in which the client's ability to make a decision is questionable. Determine the dental hygiene procedure to be performed, whether the client is able to give informed consent, the nature of their decision-making capacity, and informed refusal criteria. Finally, support your conclusion.

2. List 10 medical history questions pertaining to seizures that the dental hygiene professional must identify prior to treating the seizure disorder client.

3. Describe, in order, the steps the dental team would take to manage a seizure that occurred during treatment.

4. Role play, where one student would play the role of Thomas Small. Demonstrate how the dental hygienist would establish the professional relationship, develop a rapport, explain procedures, and answer client questions.

REFERENCES

Alvarez K: *Dental Hygiene Handbook*. Philadelphia: Lippincott Williams & Wilkins, 1999, pp. 396–398.

Bricker SL, Langlais RP, Miller CS: *Oral Diagnosis, Oral Medicine and Treatment Planning*, 2nd ed. Philadelphia: Lippincott Williams & Wilkins, 1994, pp. 30–32, 330–337, 373–380, 625–628.

Braun RJ, Cutilli BJ: *Manual of Emergency Medical Treatment for the Dental Team*. Philadelphia: Williams & Wilkins, 1999, pp. 92–94.

Darby ML, Walsh MM: *Dental Hygiene Theory and Practice*. Philadelphia: Saunders, 1994, pp. 927–942.

Gage TW, Pickett FA: *Mosby's Dental Drug Reference,* 5th ed. St. Louis: Mosby, 2001, pp. 105–106, 297–298, 534–536, 672–673.

Hodges K: *Concepts in Nonsurgical Periodontal Therapy*. Albany, NY: Delmar, 1998, pp. 17, 58.

Ibsen OAC, Phelan J: *Oral Pathology for the Dental Hygienist*, 3rd ed. Philadelphia: Saunders, 2000, pp. 64, 66, 75, 276.

Langlais RP, Miller CS: *Color Atlas of Common Oral Diseases*, 2nd ed. Philadelphia: Lippincott Williams & Wilkins, 1998, pp. 26, 50.

Little JW, Falace DA, Miller, CS, Rhodus, NL: *Dental Management of the Medically Compromised Patient*. St. Louis: Mosby, 1997, pp. 373–380.

Löe H: The gingival index, the plaque index, and the retention index systems. *Journal of Periodontology,* 38, 610–116, 1967.

Miller G, Bernstein R: *General Pathology for the Dental Hygienist*. St. Louis: Mosby, 1995, pp. 200–201, 215–233, 254–266.

Perry DA, Beemsterboer P, Taggart EJ: *Periodontology for the Dental Hygienist,* 2nd ed. Philadelphia: Saunders, 2001, pp. 53–66.

Medical Economics: *Physicians Desk Reference*, 55th ed. Montvale, NJ: Thomson Healthcare, 2001, pp. 2220–2223, 2391–2396, 2427–2430, 2458–2461.

Requa-Clark B: *Applied Pharmacology for the Dental Hygienist,* 4th ed. St. Louis: Mosby, 2000, pp, 370–376.

Weinstein B: *Informed Consent in Dental Ethics*. Philadelphia: Lea & Febiger, 1993, pp. 65–79.

Wilkins EM: *Clinical Practice of the Dental Hygienist*. Philadelphia: Lippincott Williams & Wilkins, 1999, pp. 736–760, 810–814.

Medically Compromised Client
Nancy Foster

Learning Goals

Following integration of core scientific concepts and application of dental hygiene theory to the care of this client, the student will be able to

1. **Assess client characteristics.**
   A. Recognize how diabetes effects the moisture of the oral cavity.
   B. Discriminate between the medications used for the treatment of type 1 and type 2 diabetes.
   C. Identify the classifications of diabetes using current medical terminology.
   D. Determine the etiology of the diabetes based on client history information.
   E. Recognize additional information to obtain from the client with diabetes.
   F. Relate pathophysiology of diabetes with clinical symptoms.
   G. Classify carious lesions according to G.V. Black's classification method.
   H. Identify classification of malocclusion.

2. **Obtain and interpret dental radiographs.**
   A. Identify common radiographic artifacts.
   B. Identify quality radiographic imagery.
   C. Identify normal radiographic landmarks.

3. **Plan and manage dental hygiene care.**
   A. Recognize and manage a medical emergency.
   B. Appropriately recommend recare appointment time intervals.

4. **Perform periodontal procedures.**
   A. Describe periodontal conditions.
   B. Identify periodontal risk factors.
   C. Identify the etiology of periodontal conditions.
   D. Identify the endpoint of periodontal instrumentation.

5. **Use preventive agents.**
   A. Select preventive agents based upon client needs.
   B. Determine teeth that are appropriate for pit and fissure sealant application.

6. **Provide supportive treatment services.**
   A. Recognize indications for tooth whitening procedures.

Situation

Nancy Foster is a senior in college and lives at home with her parents. She works part-time on the weekends as a waitress. A warm and friendly person, Nancy is outgoing and has plans to further her education by attending graduate school. She was diagnosed with diabetes when she was 9 years old and keeping her diabetes under control is a constant concern. She is in the office for her regular 6-month examination and prophylaxis.

For a detailed client history, including radiographs and color photos, see pages I-32 to I-33.

CLIENT'S HUMAN NEEDS DEFICITS

Because the client's oral wellness is interrelated with the client's attitudes toward health, values, and practices, and with family and cultural influences, it is important that the dental hygiene care plan be client-centered. Examination of human needs to assist the client in developing and maintaining appropriate self care reveal the following deficits:

1. Wholesome facial image

   Due to: Gingivitis and extrinsic stain
   Evidenced by: Self-report

2. Protection from health risks

   Due to: Inadequate nutrition
   Evidenced by: Self-report

3. Biologically sound and functional dentition

   Due to: Anatomy of occlusal surfaces and diet
   Evidenced by: Dental caries

4. Skin and mucous membrane integrity of the head and neck

   Due to: Presence of interproximal plaque
   Evidenced by: Gingival inflammation and bleeding

5. Responsibility for oral health

   Due to: Lack of appropriate recare interval
   Evidenced by: Gingival disease and dental caries

6. Conceptualization and understanding

   Due to: Lack of awareness of dual relationship between diabetes and oral health
   Evidenced by: Neglecting signs and symptoms of dental caries and gingival disease

QUESTIONS

Basic Questions in Assessing Client Characteristics

1. Why is xerostomia present in this client?
   A. History of orthodontic intervention
   B. Medication use

    C. Renal function
    D. Frequent meals
    E. Oral hygiene

2. Based on the current diabetes classification system by the American Diabetic Association, this client has which of the following?

    A. Type 1 diabetes
    B. Type 2 diabetes
    C. IDDM
    D. NIDDM
    E. Juvenile diabetes

3. Which of the following was the etiology in the development of this client's diabetes?

    A. Insulin resistance
    B. Inadequate insulin secretion
    C. Autoimmune destruction of β-cells
    D. Weight gain
    E. Sucrose consumption

4. Poor glycemic control may have caused this client to experience all of the following EXCEPT one. Which one is the EXCEPTION?

    A. Dental caries
    B. Dental dysplasia
    C. Increased pulse rate
    D. Weight loss
    E. Low blood pressure

5. Using G. V. Black's classification method, which of the following indicates the class of caries on the maxillary left first molar?

    A. I
    B. II
    C. III
    D. IV
    E. V

6. Which of the following MOST appropriately describes this client's molar occlusal relationship?

    A. Class I
    B. Class II, Division 1
    C. Class II, Division 2
    D. Class III

Complex Questions in Assessing Client Characteristics

7. Which question BEST elicits information about control of this client's medical condition?

    A. When was your last seizure?
    B. What is your usual blood pressure measurement?
    C. What are the results of your blood glucose testing?
    D. What year was your diabetes diagnosed?
    E. How much do you weigh?

8. Which of the following oral hypoglycemic agents is indicated considering this client's medical history?

   A. Sulfonylurea (Tolbutamide)
   B. Biguanide (Metformin)
   C. Alpha glucosidase inhibitor (Acarbose)
   D. Thiazolidinedione (Troglitazone)
   E. None of the above

Basic Questions in Obtaining and Interpreting Dental Radiographs

9. Which of the following is the most likely interpretation of the round radiolucency at the incisal edge of the mandibular right central incisor observed in the mandibular right lateral-canine periapical radiograph?

   A. Film identification dot
   B. Composite restoration
   C. Enamel pearl
   D. Calculus deposit
   E. Caries

10. Which of the following has rendered the maxillary right premolar periapical radiograph undiagnostic?

   A. Interproximal spaces overlapped
   B. Root apices not visible
   C. Cone cutting present
   D. Herringbone effect
   E. Film holder imaged

Complex Questions in Obtaining and Interpreting Dental Radiographs

11. Which of the following is the most likely interpretation of the radiolucent vertical line between the maxillary central incisors?

   A. Midpalatine suture
   B. Nutrient canal
   C. Vertical bone loss
   D. Palatal fracture
   E. Lingual foramen

Complex Questions in Planning and Managing Dental Hygiene Care

12. At her appointment today, this client seems tired and lethargic. Her skin is flushed and dry. Based on her medical history, what is your assessment?

   A. Hypoglycemia
   B. Insulin shock
   C. Insulin reaction
   D. Ketoacidosis

13. Which of the following recare appointment intervals would benefit this client?

   A. 1 month
   B. 3 months
   C. 6 months
   D. 9 months
   E. 12 months

Basic Questions in Performing Periodontal Procedures

14. Which of the following BEST describes the appearance of the facial gingiva in the region of the maxillary right central incisor?
    A. Cyanotic
    B. Erythematous
    C. Hyperkeratinized
    D. Necrotized
    E. Stippled

15. On a histologic level, which of the following is responsible for the color change of this client's gingival tissues?
    A. Collagen destruction
    B. Presence of gingival fluid
    C. Dilation of microcirculation
    D. Microulceration of the epithelium
    E. Vasostagnation of tissue fluid

Complex Questions in Performing Periodontal Procedures

16. Which of the following is the greatest risk factor for this client's periodontal disease?
    A. Blood pressure
    B. History of orthodontics
    C. Diabetes
    D. Drug side effects
    E. Xerostomia

17. What is the reason for the change in appearance of the facial gingiva in the region of the mandibular right central incisor at the 3-month recare appointment?
    A. Weight loss
    B. Medication change
    C. Scaling and root debridement
    D. Exposure to radiation
    E. Cessation of nail biting habit

Basic Question in Using Preventive Agents

18. Which of this client's molars should be indicated for pit and fissure sealants?
    A. Mandibular first molars
    B. Mandibular second molars
    C. Maxillary first molars
    D. Maxillary second molars

Complex Question in Using Preventive Agents

19. Which of the following is the BEST preventive agent to recommend to this client?
    A. End tuft toothbrush
    B. Home use fluoride
    C. Dietary assessment
    D. Tongue cleaner
    E. Automatic flosser

Complex Question in Providing Supportive Treatment Services

20. Which of the following can be expected to minimize tooth whitening results for this client?

    A. Gingival inflammation
    B. Presence of sealants
    C. Mild fluorosis
    D. Composite restoration

Answers appear on pages 97–100.

Reflective Activities

1. Since this client has little time for meal preparation with her busy schedule, develop a list of healthy foods and snacks that she could eat with little preparation.

2. Compare and contrast powered toothbrushes available on the market and identify at least two that might be appropriate to suggest for this client to improve her plaque removal.

3. Divide into groups of three to five people and discuss potential chemotherapetic agents that might be suggested to this client considering her current oral hygiene status and the clinical findings.

REFERENCES

Alvarez K: *Dental Hygiene Handbook.* Philadelphia: Williams & Wilkins, 1998, pp. 449–458.

Blackwell RE: *G.V. Black's Operative Dentistry,* Volume II, 9th ed. Milwaukee: Medico-Dental Publishing, 1955, pp. 1–4.

Darby ML, Walsh MM (eds.): *Dental Hygiene Theory and Practice.* Philadelphia: Saunders, 1994, pp. 913–925.

Gerlach RW: Shifting paradigms in whitening: Introduction of a novel system for vital tooth bleaching. Supplement to *Compendium of Continuing Education in Dentistry,* 21 (suppl.), S5, S8, 2000.

Haring JI, Lind LJ: *Radiographic Interpretation for the Dental Hygienist.* Philadelphia: Saunders, 1993, pp. 25–58.

Hodges K: *Concepts in Nonsurgical Periodontal Therapy.* Albany, NY: Delmar, 1997, pp. 88–117.

Ibsen OAC, Phelan J: *Oral Pathology for the Dental Hygienist,* 3rd ed. Philadelphia: Saunders, 2000, p. 46.

Kinane DF: Periodontitis mediated by systemic factors. *Annals of Periodontology,* 4, 54–55, 1999.

Little JW, Falace DA: *Dental Management of the Medically Compromised Patient.* St. Louis: Mosby, 1993, pp. 387–409.

Löe H: The gingival index, the plaque index, and the retention index systems. *Journal of Periodontology,* 38, 610–616, 1967.

Nizel A, Papas A: *Nutrition in Clinical Dentistry,* 3rd ed. Philadelphia: Saunders, 1989, pp. 25–28.

Murphy IP: Bleaching wins acceptance as a treatment of choice. *Access,* 10, M-22, 1996.

Slavkin HC: Diabetes, clinical dentistry and changing paradigms. *Journal of the American Dental Association,* 128(5), 638–644, 1997.

Wilkins EM: *Clinical Practice of the Dental Hygienist,* 8th ed. Philadelphia: Lippincott Williams & Wilkins, 1999, pp. 235, 252, 482, 880–891.

ANSWERS AND RATIONALES

CASE A

1. **D** The scalloped appearance of the incisal edges of the anterior teeth is characteristic of mamelons, developmental lobes found on the incisal edges of newly erupted teeth. *Perikymata* refers to horizontal developmental lines seen on the facial surface of some anterior teeth. Enamel hypoplasia appears as pitting in the enamel surface, whereas mild fluorosis appears as a white "snow capping" along the incisal edges of anterior teeth. Attrition appears as the wearing away of the incisal edge as a result of contact with the teeth of the opposing arch. In fact, over time, this contact will result in the attrition of the mamelons.

2. **C** The dorsal surface of this client's tongue appears to have a yellow coating indicating a need for oral self-care instruction in tongue cleaning. This appearance should not be mistaken for a disease state such as lymphangioma, which would manifest in enlarged lymphoid aggregates. Lymphangioma appears as a raised yellow-pink swelling frequently located on the lateral posterior of the tongue. A fissured tongue occurs infrequently in children, and is often considered a condition of aging. Additionally, the tongue does not appear to be enlarged (macroglossia) or ulcerated.

3. **C** The cusp of the mandibular permanent first premolar appears to be erupting into its appropriate position in the arch. The radiographic appearance of this area confirms this clinical assessment.

4. **C** Her pulse rate is considered high. The following arc considered within normal limits for children: pulse rate for a 10-year-old child is 70 bpm; respiration for an 8-year-old child is 20 bpm; mean blood pressure for a 6-year-old child is 114/74 mm Hg and 122/78 mm Hg for a 12-year-old child.

5. **B** She is most likely exhibiting signs of apprehension and tension in anticipation of her dental treatment today. The nervous client typically presents with an increased pulse rate, dry mouth and shortness of breath. These symptoms may also be side effects of the Albuterol and Claritin. Additionally, the clinician should watch and listen carefully to recognize the presence of anxiety and to prepare for the possibility of an asthma attack.

6. **E** This client's gingival bleeding is a result of bacterial plaque accumulation and is not a side effect of Albuterol and Claritin.

7. **E** The radiopacity seen above the maxillary teeth is the hard palate. The incisive foramen, nasal fossae, and median palatine suture would all appear as radiolucencies. The nasal septum would appear

radiopaque, but is imaged as a vertical radiopacity between the maxillary central incisors.

8. **C** This client has an exaggerated gag reflex that makes it difficult to place film intraorally. While it is true that a fast film and lower dosage of radiation is used, a panoramic radiograph enabled the clinician to manage the client's behavior.

9. **A** When an object is positioned outside of the panoramic focal trough, or the imaginary zone of sharpness, the object will not be imaged on the film. The natural tilt of the anterior teeth in the arches places the apices of these teeth outside the focal trough, causing the tooth roots to not be imaged on the film. This phenomenon of panoramic imaging should not be mistaken for external physiologic resorption or incomplete root formation. *Microdontia* refers to a tooth that develops at a smaller size than normal.

10. **A** Brushing the tongue is the recommended daily oral hygiene instruction for this client. Tongue scraping, although often recommended, may be more difficult for a child of this age level and manual dexterity. Daily oral rinses do not debride the tongue and oral irrigation is recommended for cleansing subgingivally. Breath freshener tablets will not remove microorganisms from the tongue.

11. **C** Power-driven polishing instruments are contraindicated for the client who presents with asthma. Additionally, the client who presents with xerostomia cannot afford to have the fluoride rich enamel surface weakened by polishing. Because this client has moderate accumulations of stain, scaling followed by a toothbrushing with an over-the-counter toothpaste is indicated.

12. **D** The client should be placed in a comfortable position to ease breathing. A comfortable position almost always involves sitting, with the arms forward. The Trendelenberg position with the feet elevated 10 to 15 degrees is used to increase blood flow to the brain as in vasodepressor syncope; it is contraindicated in this situation. Given this client's medical history, an asthma attack may become evident, at which time she should be administered a bronchodilator The clinician should discontinue any treatment and provide verbal reassurance to this client.

13. **A** Tell, show, do as a child management technique is the simplest and most effective way to handle children. Oral sedation would be an extreme measure for managing this client. Additionally, adding another drug to this child client's current medications may not be prudent. Papoose board restriction is used to control physical movements for a client who may be spastic or unruly. Hypnosis and biofeedback are management techniques generally used for adult dental phobic clients.

14. **C** These three species of bacteria have strong association in the etiology of gingivitis observed in this client. *Streptococcus salivaris* is usually found in high proportions on the tongue and in the saliva and is less concentrated on the teeth. *Fusobacterium nucleatum* and *Prevotella intermedia* are associated with refractory chronic periodontitis, while *Actinobacillus actinomycetemcomitans* has a strong association in the etiology of localized juvenile periodontitis. *Streptococcus mutans* and lactobaccilli are the etiologic bacteria in dental caries.

15. **D** The rounded toe, curved back, and complex shank of the universal curet allows for subgingival instrumentation in shallow pockets. A flexible shank would be used to remove light deposits throughout the mouth. This one instrument could be used to increase time efficiency, whereas the area-specific Gracey curets would require the clinician to constantly change instruments to complete the whole mouth. The sickle scalers are not the best choice due to design characteristics such as pointed tip, triangular working end, and straight lateral surfaces. Ultrasonic scalers are contraindicated on primary teeth and light calculus.

16. **D** The primary molars do not have developmental pits in the occlusal anatomy and would not need sealant placement. Also, according to the radiographic interpretation, these teeth will be exfoliated soon. The permanent premolars and permanent second molars have not erupted.

17. **B** The use of xerostomia-causing medications puts this client at an increased risk for caries; therefore, a fluoride rinse is the most appropriate choice.

18. **B** Neutral sodium fluoride is the agent of choice for clients with reduced salivary flow. Although acidulated phosphate fluoride (APF) provides rapid and high fluoride uptake in the enamel, its high acidity contraindicates its use for this client with xerostomia. Stannous is rarely used today as a professional topical fluoride application. Sodium monofluorophosphate is a fluoride preparation found in dentifrice, and is not used for professional applications.

19. **C** This client's medications do not interfere with nutrient absorption or utilization. All the remaining factors are important considerations for nutritional counseling. The amounts and frequency of eating fermentable carbohydrates has the greatest potential for decay and may be a factor in cultural food preference and eating habits. Understanding this risk potential for caries and explaining the importance of a well balanced diet from all food groups would be important nutritional counseling information to share with the preparer of the child's food.

20. **C** This client presents with an exaggerated gag reflex that can be anticipated to make impressions difficult to take. While sensitive gingiva might be a client complaint, this is not a general contraindication for impressions. Frenal attachments and occlusal articulation should not cause problems in achieving a good impression.

CASE B

1. **C** The client's facial profile is best described as retrognathic. Although usually associated with a Class II category of Angle's classification of occlusion (and this client exhibits a Class I category), the client's chin appears retruded, giving the mandible a small appearance. Contributing further to a retrognathic profile, to keep the lips closed at rest, this client presents with an unbalanced facial musculature. The decreased maxillary lip thickness is indicative of obvious lip strain to achieve a lip seal at occlusal rest. Mesiognathic and orthognathic profiles are demonstrated by a harmonious facial profile in which the maxilla and mandible appear balanced and the lips seal lightly at occlusal rest without muscle strain. Usually associated with a Class III category of Angle's classification of occlusion, a prognathic profile appears as a

reverse of the retrognathic profile, i.e., the chin appears protruded, giving the mandible a larger or longer appearance when compared with the maxilla.

2. **A** Angle's classification of occlusion is determined by the relationship of the permanent maxillary and mandibular first molars. If the mesiobuccal cusp of the permanent maxillary first molar occludes in line with the buccal groove of the permanent mandibular first molar, the occlusion is deemed "normal." In addition to the permanent first molar relationship, the permanent maxillary and mandibular canines and the relationship of the anterior teeth can be used to determine a Class I malocclusion. In the Class I malocclusion, exhibited by this client, the anterior teeth present with crowding, a significant overjet, and moderate to severe overbite. If the buccal groove of the permanent mandibular first molar aligns distal to the mesiobuccal cusp of the permanent maxillary first molar, then Class II malocclusion is demonstrated. The relationship between the anterior teeth is used to determine the two subdivisions of a Class II malocclusion. Division 1 is demonstrated when the maxillary anterior teeth occlude facially in relationship with the mandibular anterior teeth. Division 2 is demonstrated when the one of more of the maxillary anterior teeth occlude lingually in relationship with the mandibular anterior teeth. If the buccal groove of the permanent mandibular first molar aligns mesial to the mesiobuccal cusp of the permanent maxillary first molar, then Class III malocclusion is demonstrated.

3. **C** The physiologic external root resorption evident on the primary left second molar viewed in the panoramic radiograph indicates that this tooth will be exfoliated next. While the primary maxillary left second molar also exhibits physiologic external root resorption, it appears less extensive. Additionally, the maxillary teeth usually follow the mandibular teeth in a normal exfoliation and eruption pattern. The exfoliated primary left second molar will be replaced by the developing permanent left second premolar viewed in the panoramic radiograph.

4. **D** The most likely cause of this client's nocturnal bruxism is occlusal interference. Malocclusion may cause grinding or clenching outside the normal range of chewing. Because this client is undergoing orthodontic treatment, his occlusion is in transition and discrepancies in centric occlusion and centric relation is thought to be a cause of noctural bruxism.

5. **A** The radiographs indicate that all of this client's permanent teeth are present and developing normally. Additionally, there are no congenitally missing teeth or supernumerary teeth evident. However, the permanent maxillary and mandibular first molar and canine relationships indicate an Angle's Class I malocclusion, with significant anterior crowding.

6. **D** Fluorosis can be described as areas on the teeth of parchment white color representing hypocalcification of tooth enamel. This client's history of exposure to high a concentration of fluoride during tooth development further indicates the possibility of fluorosis.

7. **E** Buccal pit amalgam restorations are visible in the photographs of this client. Furthermore, because of the dense nature of amalgam, these restorations will appear radiopaque on the resultant radio-

graphs. The location, size, shape, and margin of these radiopacities indicate the presence of amalgam restorations on these teeth.

8. **A** Cephalometric radiographs are most often used to evaluate growth and development and are especially useful in the assessment for orthodontic intervention and treatment.

9. **C** A cephalometric radiograph utilizes a cephalostat or head holder to stabilize the client in position. The cephalostat employs the use of two plastic ear rods. To stabilize the skull into position and to provide a basis for standardization of subsequent radiographs, one plastic ear rod is inserted into each ear. As the x-ray beam penetrates the cephalostat, a portion of the beam is blocked by the ear rods, leaving less x rays to strike the film. The resultant image is a radiopaque object resembling the shape of the ear rods.

10. **B** Proper positioning for cephalometric radiographs requires the location and alignment of skeletal landmarks. The Frankfort plane or orbitomeatal line, which extends from the superior border of the external auditory meatus to the infraorabital rim is an important reference line when positioning the client for cephalometric radiographs. The forehead positioner of the cephalostat is the object visible in this radiograph.

11. **D** The developing tooth first appears radiographically as a round or oval radiolucency. The cusps begin to calcify first, followed by the root. The root continues to develop throughout the eruption process. While the crown of a tooth may appear to be completely erupted, the root may still be developing. As the root develops, the pulp chamber appears to narrow and close at the apex. Additionally, until development is completed, the soft tissue forming the root, dentinal papillae may be seen as a radiolucency at the apex of the tooth.

12. **C** Clients this age and their friends are often misinformed regarding the relationship of spit tobacco and athletic performance. While this client most likely receives an abundance of health information, the media and althletic role models often impress children and adolescents with misinformation. However, in a major league baseball poll, not one player who used dip or spit tobacco said that the tobacco improved his game or sharpened his reflexes. Adolescents are aware that spit tobacco is highly addictive, and are usually informed that a user will absorb more nicotine from spit tobacco than from cigarettes.

13. **A** Effective toothbrushing is this client's greatest immediate need. Because he hates to brush around his braces, an automatic toothbrush would be an effective plaque removal alternative to the manual brush. An oral irrigation device is recommended as a useful adjunct to toothbrushing, but this client's primary problem must first be addressed. Oral irrigation can be added later once brushing effectiveness is achieved. Floss threaders and the use of a sulcus brush are time consuming. Motivation to use additional self-care aids will be possible in the future if the dental hygienist can first reinforce this client's plaque removal success with the automatic toothbrush.

14. **B** Children as young as 5 should be asked about their use of tobacco. If they are not using the drug they should be congratulated for positive health behaviors to reinforce and increase the likelihood of continuing

this behavior. Initiation of tobacco use is highly correlated in the adolescent age group as a result of the insecurity and rebellious characteristics of this age group. Media stereotypes and star athletes are powerful influences in teenagers' behaviors and self-image.

15. **E** Convincing adolescents to accept and comply with preventive regimens is difficult due to their orientation to present time activities and lack of concern for preventive health care in general. Discussion of developing important health habits for the future, such as the need for orthodontic intervention, protection from risks of athletic activities, and tobacco cessation programs, may not seem pertinent to youth in this age group. Characteristics of this age group that can be constructively used for positive health behaviors include: fully developed sense of logic, increasing independence from parental influence, sense of reality and conceptualization of the scientific principles of cause and effect.

16. **C** Although adolescents generally possess the dexterity to perform a self-care regime that will maintain their oral health, they typically lack the motivation to perform these skills on a regular basis. First, appealing to their perceived needs motivates them to act on new, healthy behaviors. Secondly, providing a new or unique oral hygiene aid that appeals to the adolescent, such as a fashionable toothbrush, can provide an additional motivator to perform the desired healthy behaviors. Because adolescents are striving for independence from parental control, parents of adolescents play a very minimal role in oral self care of these clients.

17. **B** *Festooning* refers to marginal gingiva that appears enlarged and rolled. Moderate festooning can appear as a doughnut-shaped ring of gingiva around the teeth.

18. **A** During the eruption of the teeth, the appearance of the gingiva is often described as thickened, rounded, or rolled. As the eruption process continues, the gingival appearance flattens out and the marginal gingiva takes on a more knifelike appearance. This can be observed when comparing this client's photographs one month later.

19. **C** This client's teeth are indicated for air-powder abrasive polishing to effectively remove plaque and stain around his orthodontic appliances. Because he has his permanent dentition and no respiratory illnesses this procedure is not contraindicated for this method of stain removal. Rubber cup polishing would be difficult around the orthodontic brackets and may not be completely effective at stain removal. Although time consuming, the port polisher and the manual toothbrush are effective devices when professional powered stain removal techniques are contraindicated.

20. **D** Because the Academy of Sports Dentistry recommends mouth protection for clients who skateboard, this client should be using a mouth protector specifically designed for adolescents who engage in sports and/or recreational activities that increase the risk for trauma to the oral cavity. A thermoplastic boil-and-bite mouth protector is the appropriate appliance choice for a client in orthodontic brackets. A hard plastic thermoset resin mouthguard is used to treat adult nocturnal bruxism and would not be indicated for this client.

CASE C

1. **A** G.V. Black established the standard for classifying caries in the early 1900s. This system has since been customarily used for describing cavity preparations and restorations as well. The amalgam restoration observed on the lingual surface of the maxillary left lateral incisor is classified as a Class I restoration. Class I restorations involve only one surface of the tooth, such as the occlusal surface only of posterior teeth; facial and lingual surface only of molars; and/or the lingual surface only of incisors. Class II restorations were not included as an option. Class III restorations involve proximal surfaces of incisors and canines that do not involve the incisal angle, where as Class IV restorations do involve the incisal angle. Class V restorations are placed along the cervical one third of facial and lingual surfaces (not pits or fissures). Class VI restorations involve incisal edges of anterior teeth and cusp tips of posterior teeth.

2. **D** As seen in the photographs, preparations have been made on the distal portions of the occlusal surfaces of the maxillary second premolars for the removable partial denture clasp rest that is positioned on the abutment teeth to support the partial denture. The maxillary anterior teeth support the major connector. The mandibular left posterior teeth are restored with a fixed partial denture that is not removable. The maxillary first molars are missing and replaced by the pontics of the removable partial denture.

3. **E** Life-long residence in a community with near-optimal levels of water fluoridation reduces the incidence of root caries 30% as compared with communities with nonfluoridated water supplies. This client also uses fluoride rinses along with her dentifrice. Prosthetic devices and restorations provide plaque retentive areas. A history of many coronal restorations indicate an increased risk for root caries. Xerostomia is a side effect of the medications taken by this client. Gingival recession is necessary for root surface caries as it exposes the cemental surface to mutans streptococcus and lactobacilli as the primary organisms associated with root caries. The oral photographs reveal plaque accumulation in the mandibular anterior region as supported by the appearance of gingival redness.

4. **B** The radiographs reveal the presence of retention pins, which are distinguished from the other materials by their size and shape. Additionally, a post-and-core restoration and silver points and gutta percha endodontic filling materials would appear to penetrate the pulp chamber and root canals.

5. **D** A radiopaque appearance indicates no exposure to radiographs. In this case the metal arm of a film holding device appears to have blocked a portion of the x-ray beam, leaving the area directly behind the device unexposed. While a metal clasp of a partial denture would produce a similar appearance, the clasp would not appear in this area. While metal scraps from amalgam also will block the x-ray beam and leave a radiopaque appearance on the image, an amalgam fragment, which embeds in the gingiva, would not appear on the edge of the film in this manner or size. Additionally, cone cut error would be more uniform in appearance representing the edge of the position indicating device (PID).

6. **E** Radiographically, the slightly increased radiopacity visible on the distal and occlusal surfaces of the mandibular right second premolar indicates the presence of a composite restoration. The significantly increased radiopacity of the material present on the maxillary right first premolar and the maxillary left first premolar indicates amalgam restorations. The smooth margins of the restorations present on the mandibular left first premolar and the maxillary left second premolar indicate metal crowns.

7. **A** The classic appearance of the mental foramen is a round or oval radiolucency located near the mandibular first or second premolar. This radiolucency should not be confused with apical pathology.

8. **B** Assessing whether the crestal bone is parallel with the cemento-enamel junctions (CEJs) of the adjacent teeth determines horizontal bone loss. The distal aspect of the mandibular first molar exhibits vertical bone loss because an imaginary line drawn across the height of the crestal bone is not parallel with an imaginary line drawn connecting the CEJs of the two molars. Horizontal bone loss is evident on most of this client's other teeth as the crestal bone is parallel with a line connecting the CEJs on the adjacent teeth. Periodontal abscesses are seen as large diffuse radiolucencies in a lateral position to the tooth. Furcation involvement would appear as a radiolucency between the roots.

9. **C** Given this client's history of syncope and ischemic heart disease, care should be taken to provide a stress-free environment to avoid a fainting episode or the onset of an angina attack. Warmth and caring demonstrated by the dental professional can reduce the risk of one of these emergencies. A semisupine chair position is recommended for clients with angina pectoris. Allowing time for adjustment to change in chair position may help to avoid orthostatic hypotension of which the occurrence is an increased side effect of the drug Cardizem. The dental professional can further avoid an emergency situation by requiring that the client bring the nitroglycerine to the appointment in case an attack was to occur. Additionally, having ammonia capsules available would allow the dental professional to arouse an unconscious client, thus avoiding a more serious situation. This client does not present with a need for antibiotic prophylaxis.

10. **B** A therapy regimen that includes segmental scaling and root debridement, especially when anesthesia is used to increase client comfort, improves success. Therefore this client would benefit from having two shorter appointments for scaling and root debridement. Clients completing nonsurgical periodontal therapy should be scheduled for 3-month recare intervals for the first year following therapy to allow frequent evaluation of the periodontal status. Clients on 3-month intervals experience less disease progression and less loss of attachment. Area specific Gracey curets are the hand instruments of choice for debridement because the complex shank allows access to the root surfaces whereas universal instruments have limited access. Selective polishing with the rubber cup method is the approach recommended for clients with periodontal diseases because it supports client self-care and the goals of professional therapy, therefore air abrasive polishing would be contraindicated for this client. Additionally this client may be on a salt-restricted diet due to her heart condition.

11. **E** Vital signs such as blood pressure may be an indicator of a client's anxiety levels not the cause. In this case the client presents with a history of past dental experiences that involved pain where her response was fainting. It is therefore expected that these past experiences will be effected by her response to today's visit. Additionally, this client's need to be self-reliant may be adding to her overly enthusiastic apprehension regarding her ability to control her reactions to treatment. Also, the side effects of the drug Voltran include an increase in anxiety levels.

12. **D** Age, hormonal therapies, history of periodontal disease, as evidenced by recession and stress, have all been identified as risk factors for periodontal disease. Drug allergies are not associated with increased risk for periodontal breakdown thus tetracycline allergy is not a risk factor.

13. **D** The clinical attachment level is determined by the probe depth and assessment of the position of the gingival margin in relation to a fixed point, the CEJ. When recession is present, the attachment loss is equal to the amount of recession plus the periodontal probe depth reading. With 4 mm of recession and a 2 mm facial probing depth the loss of attachment would be 6 mm in this area.

14. **E** Mucogingival involvement is determined by measuring the width of attached gingiva and subtracting the periodontal probe reading. When the resulting measurement is less than 1 mm there is mucogingival involvement. The mandibular right lateral incisor exhibits apparent recession that has progressed almost to the mucogingival line. With an average 2 mm pocket depth, this area is most at risk for mucogingival involvement. The other teeth do not have as much recession and thus are at less risk.

15. **E** The mandibular right first molar is a candidate for local drug delivery with an 8 mm pocket that did not decrease at the 6-month recare appointment. Because this area did not positively respond to mechanical therapy, and the possibility exists that periodontal surgery is not always an option for all clients, local drug delivery should be an optional treatment. The other teeth do not have sufficient pocket depths for placement of local drug treatment.

16. **C** Because the client is allergic to tetracycline, chlorhexidine chip delivery method is the correct response. All of the other agents contain derivatives of tetracycline as their active ingredient.

17. **D** Potassium nitrate is the active ingredient found in at-home-use toothpaste with the American Dental Asociation (ADA) seal for treatment of hypersensitive teeth. All of the other chemical agents are found in professional treatments rather than self-applied agents available for homecare.

18. **B** Postmenopausal women on estrogen replacement therapies are at greater risk for dental caries due to a decrease in salivary flow. Although this client leaves plaque in the mandibular anterior facial area, compliance with plaque control, following instruction is expected to be high. Tooth/host resistance seems adequate with this client's history of community water fluoridation. In addition, there was no indication of high frequency of sucrose intake in the information provided by the client.

19. **C** Because reduction of pain is mandatory for the successful management of the client with ischemic heart disease and significantly sensitive root surfaces, this client requires deep local anesthesia to provide pulpal and soft tissue comfort during treatment. This is achieved through injection lidocaine (Xylocaine) and not topical applications such as topical benzocaine or the use of a transoral method (Dentipatch). While nitrous oxide sedation and orally ingesting 2 to 5 mg of diazepam will highly reduce the client's stress and anxiety, these drugs will not be successful in providing the deep anesthesia required to complete root debridement.

20. **A** Nightguard therapy is recommended to reduce the parafunctional habit of nocturnal bruxism and will resolve the tooth mobility due to decreased functional demand. An additional expected outcome of this therapy would be arrested periodontal destruction in the area. Biofeedback and therapeutic massage will help the client reduce bruxism but will not provide tooth mobility treatment. Splinting the teeth will provide stabilization of tooth mobility; however, it does not eliminate the bruxism and attrition that will continue to occur.

CASE D

1. **B** *Leukoplakia* is the term given to white patches found intraorally that usually cannot be clinically identified as a specific disease entity. While smoking may have initiated the epithelium in this area to increase in thickness, trauma created by movement of the upper lip over this tissue could also produce the hyperkeratinization. The etiology may not be readily discernable and a histological exam may be ordered for differential diagnosis. Luekodema, Fordyce's granules, nicotinic stomatitis, and candidiasis can usually be distinguished by their characteristic appearances and the location in which they are noted. Luekodema, found in approximately 80% of the black population, appears as a milky, white-blue striated lesion of the buccal mucosa, and Fordyce's granules, subaceous glands choristomas, appear more yellow in color and are usually found near the maxillary vermilion border and labial mucosa. Both are considered normal conditions and no treatment is necessary. Nicotinic stomatitis can result in hyperkeratosis of the mucosa of the hard palate in response to the heat introduced into the oral cavity from smoking. The palate usually appears white with small red points. Candidiasis, representing the overgrowth of *Candida albicans,* which may result when the normal flora of the oral cavity is altered as when the client is taking antibiotics, is immune suppressed, presents with endocrine diseases or has a hereditary predisposition to fungal infections. In the case of pseudomembranous candidiasis, this white lesion may be easily wiped off with a gauze sponge.

2. **B** Overjet, underjet, and anterior crossbite refer to the horizontal distance between the labioincisal surfaces of the maxillary anterior teeth and the lingualoincisal surfaces of the mandibular anterior teeth. When overjet presents, the maxillary anterior teeth are in a position labial to the mandibular anterior teeth, whereas when underjet and/or anterior crossbite present, the maxillary anterior teeth are in a position lingual to the mandibular anterior teeth. In an edge-to-edge relationship, the anterior teeth occlude on the incisal edge, whereas an open

bite indicates a lack of contact (vertical opening) between the maxillary and mandibular anterior teeth.

3. **A** Normal melanin pigmentation occurs in people of color and should not be mistakenly identified as a disease or condition requiring attention.

4. **C** The maxillary frenum functions to hold the lip in place. The size and location of the labial frenal attachment may effect the position of the maxillary central incisors laterally. This band of connective tissue is so firm that erupting central incisors may not penetrate through it, but will be pushed aside so that a diastema may result. While a growing cyst or tumor may indeed displace structures in its path, the radiolucency between the maxillary central incisors is the incisive foramen and should not be mistaken for a pathologic condition. Additionally, destruction of bone and the development of infrabony defects as the result of periodontal disease, will cause tooth mobility and displacement. However, probe depths and radiographic assessment of the maxillary central incisors do not reveal conditions conducive to distal drift of these teeth. While the client does present with a tongue thrust, this condition may be contributing to his pronounced over jet through forces inflicted anteriorly, but not the diastema which is the result of forces inflicted laterally. The enlarged papilla, unlike the frenal attachment, is not involved in mechanical movement and therefore would not be exerting force on the tooth structure to cause displacement.

5. **D** The incisive foramen is anatomically located between the maxillary central incisors. Of this list of foramina, only the incisive and infraorbital will appear on a maxillary radiograph. Because of its superior location, the infraorbital foramen may be imaged on a panoramic radiograph, but not on an intra oral radiograph. The mental foramen and lingual foramen may appear on mandibular periapical radiographs, while the mandibular foramen, because of its posterior/superior location in the ramus of the mandible, may appear on a panoramic radiograph, but not on an intraoral radiograph.

6. **B** Calculus appears about the radiopacity of dentin and may be visible as a "bump" or spur on the proximal surface of the tooth or between the teeth and/or roots of the tooth. In cases of gross deposits, calculus may appear as a band or clump across the tooth. While an enamel pearl may present in this area between the roots, it would appear the same radiopacity as enamel and would be attached to, or appear as an extension of the enamel. Pulp stones present within the pulp chamber and hypercementosis would appear as an overgrowth of excess cementum creating an enlarged or bulbous root structure. Composite restorations would not be placed in this area and would appear in a prepared cavity within the tooth structure rather than an "attachment" to the root.

7. **D** This client reports that he recently began using an automatic toothbrush. His technique with this device should be evaluated versus teaching him new methods and aids.

8. **D** To help the client meet his goals of improving oral health and to encourage success of non-surgical periodontal intervention, the first step must be client education in the disease process and explicit instruction in oral self care. The success of periodontal maintenance depends on

the role the client plays in oral self-care on a daily basis, therefore prior to any therapeutic intervention, instruction in oral self-assessment and discussion of the relationship between preventive measures and periodontal disease must occur.

9. **B** Premature loss of mandibular teeth may result in the hypereruption of the opposing maxillary teeth. While furcation involvement is present, it is the result, and not the cause of the hypereruption of the maxillary molars. Neither would the remaining conditions cause the hypereruption.

10. **A** The Nabors probe contains markings to gage the depth of penetration through the furcation area of periodontally involved teeth.

11. **B** Gracey curets are site specific scaling and root planing instruments. The 11/12 Gracey curet is designed specifically for instrumentation of the mesial surfaces of posterior teeth. Gracey curets are especially useful in deep, nonaccessible periodontal pockets.

12. **C** Horizontal bone loss is differentiated from a vertical or angular defect by comparing the bone crest to an imaginary line draw from cementoenamel junctions (CEJ) of adjacent teeth. When the alveolar bone crest appears parallel to the imaginary line draw from cementoenamel junctions of adjacent teeth then horizontal bone loss is noted. When an opening or "window" appears through the bone covering the facial root surface, the condition is referred to as fenestration, whereas when this opening or loss of bone manifests in a resorbed cleft, the condition is dehiscence, neither of which are associated with these teeth.

13. **C** In the 1950s, Glickman developed the classification of furcation involvement identified by grades. Significant bone loss in the furcation area in which the bone is not attached to the dome of the furcation and the probe may pass through the roots is classified as a Grade III. If the soft tissues have receded apically so that the furcation is clinically visible, Grade IV is the appropriate classification, (but this was not one of the answer choices). The classification is a Grade II furcation when there is horizontal and vertical bone loss essentially creating a cul-de-sac; radiographs may or may not depict the involvement. Grade I furcation involvement is early bone destruction where radiographic changes are not evident.

14. **B** Eight millimeters is the distance from the exposed CEJ to the attached tissue at the base of the clinical pocket. The amount of recession, 3 mm as indicated by the probe, is added to the probing depth to yield the clinical attachment level. Normal clinical attachment level is located at the CEJ.

15. **D** The concave root morphology on the mesial surface of the maxillary first premolar provides a protected environment for bacteria to accumulate. While the other conditions—overhanging restorations, caries, and occlusal trauma—may be risk factors for periodontal disease, these conditions are not evident in this area. This tooth has under gone endodontic therapy; however, this procedure is limited to the pulp chamber and does not have an implication in periodontal disease.

16. **A** While tooth mobility may result from various conditions, such as trauma or periapical pathology, only one of the conditions listed in the question is responsible for this client's tooth mobility. The significant

bone loss associated with periodontal disease exhibited by this client is responsible for the mobile teeth.

17. **C** It has been established that tobacco smoking may be the most important environmental factor in the U.S. associated with periodontal disease. The exact mechanisms are unknown, but evidence exists that points to smoking's effect on peripheral blood production and alteration in peripheral blood immunioregulatory T cells.

18. **D** The effects and benefits of nonsurgical debridement include all of the possible responses to this question, however, the photographs demonstrate no change in the locations of the gingival margin, color or gingival consistency. When the photographs are compared with the probing depths, the clinician is left to conclude that the actual outcome of debridement is a long junctional epithelial attachment rather than tissue shrinkage or complete regeneration of the connective tissue.

19. **A** Because nicotine addiction is so difficult to overcome, positive reinforcement and complimenting the client on his success so far can often be an impetus to continued success. Likewise, slipping, or smoking again, can be very discouraging to the client trying to quit. Making the client aware that he can try to stop again, and has not "failed," if he smokes one or a few cigarettes, can provide needed motivation. To get the maximum benefit from nicotine gum, the client may need to be reminded of the instructions on its use. Nicotine gum should be used whenever the urge to smoke occurs. Nicotine gum should be chewed slowly for 30 minutes and then "parked" inside the cheek against the oral mucosa. Every few minutes, he may repeat slow, gentle chewing. Overcoming nicotine addiction can be especially difficult in the beginning, since it may take 1 or 2 weeks for withdrawal symptoms to subside. Providing the client with this information along with encouragement and support from the dental hygienist will aid in his success.

20. **B** Because past periodontal disease creates an increased risk for future destruction, an increased schedule for periodontal maintenance procedures in recommended. Currently, based on the assessment of this client, most studies indicate a 3-month periodontal maintenance procedure schedule.

CASE E

1. **D** An amalgam tattoo presents on the lingual of the maxillary right first molar when viewing the intraoral photographs. Amalgam tattoos appear as a localized gray-blue discoloration due to the inadvertent depositing of amalgam fragments into the gingiva during the tooth preparation.

2. **D** This bony projection in the midline of the palate is the typical appearance of a torus palantinus and should not be confused with pathosis or conditions requiring further diagnosis.

3. **E** Abfraction lesions occur when mechanical stress of teeth is exceeded during mastication. The maxillary first and second molars have porcelain fused to metal crowns that exert loading pressure on the mandibular teeth which creates flexure at the cervix. Repeated flexing

results in loss of tooth structure on the buccal surfaces of the cervical one third of the tooth.

4. **B** While age and occlusal trauma may exacerbate gingival recession, this client's gingival recession is the result of periodontal disease. Gingival recession is contributing to the root caries process due to exposure of the cementum in the oral cavity.

5. **C** TMJ dysfunction may be found in 45% to 75% of arthritic clients. Symptoms include pain, stiffness, swelling, and decreased mobility.

6. **A** The radiopaque appearance of the pulp chambers of this tooth indicate the presence of endodontic filling material and rule out observing pulpstones. Instead, gutta percha and a post-and-core restoration can be observed on the radiograph of this tooth. The spiral pin core is similar in appearance to an endosseous implant; however, the tooth root is still visible indicating that this restorative material is not an implant. The length and morphology of the root indicates no resorption or apicoectomy.

7. **E** The technique error evidenced on the maxillary right canine periapical radiograph is cone cutting. Cone cutting is corrected by completely covering the film with the x-ray beam so that the entire radiograph is exposed. In this case, it is the inferior portion of the radiograph that did not get exposed. The PID should be moved inferiorly to completely expose the film.

8. **A** Vertical bitewing radiographs provide increased imaging in the vertical dimension over horizontal bitewings, which is especially valuable for use in the periodontally involved client. This increased visibility allows imaging of significant bone loss. However, vertical placement of the bitewing radiograph does not provide information about the apices of teeth and therefore would not replace periapical radiographs. The presence of large tori and TMD which make opening painful or difficult may interfere with film packet placement and actually hinder the use of vertical bitewings. The client's age plays no role in the orientation of the film packet.

9. **C** The mandibular right lateral incisor appears to have been extensively restored. Given the history of restorative trauma to this tooth, the rounded radiolucency observed at the apex of this tooth should be suspected to be indicative of a periapical abscess. While the mental foramen would also appear as a round radiolucency, the foramen would not be located in this area. Genial tubercles and tori appear radiopaque and do not resemble the finding noted in the question. Additionally, the film identification dot should not be confused as an interpretive finding.

10. **B** Coumadin interferes with blood clotting which may lead to excessive bleeding following scaling. Therefore, a medical consult should determine this client's prothrombin time or international normalized ratio (INR) status prior to proceeding with scaling. The coumadin dose may need to be reduced or stopped just prior to scaling to prevent excessive bleeding.

11. **B** Clients taking a diuretic to manage hypertension are often advised to limit the use of sodium-containing products. This client is taking the diuretic chlorthiazide (Diuril). Therefore, air-powder abrasive polishing, which uses sodium bicarbonate, would be contraindicated.

12. **E** Effective communication for the client with a history of a stroke requires good communicative techniques that include speaking clearly and slowly, directly to the client; frequent feedback to make sure that the client comprehends what is being communicated; and the use of basic, uncomplicated media. It is also important that the client's abilities are neither underestimated nor overestimated. Often the healthcare professional is careful about not underestimating abilities of the individual. However, stroke victims are often unaware of the extent of their paresis. Therefore, it is important that the dental hygienist not overestimate the client's abilities, and take a proactive stance with the stroke-prone client and provide assistance when seating or dismissing the client or changing chair positions.

13. **E** This client's osteoarthritis is causing morning stiffness in his hips and knees, which makes it difficult for him to walk. A later appointment would allow the stiffness to dissipate and increase his ambulatory capabilities.

14. **C** This client's arthritis is the likely cause of his TMD. Treatment and recommendations including a soft diet, application of moist heat, and fabrication of an occlusal appliance, can be undertaken at his oral healthcare facility without the prescription of a physician.

15. **C** This client's probing depths indicate a moderate periodontal disease state in the posterior regions. When probe-depth readings of the anterior teeth are combined with the the amount of recession in these regions, the total loss of attachment indicates a moderate periodontal disease state. Therefore, this client's periodontal status is considered generalized.

16. **E** While this client attributes his health to his faith, an examination of his oral cavity reveals extensive past dental treatment indicating that he does not appear to object to oral healthcare by professionals.

17. **C** Placing this client on a 6-month recare appointment schedule would be inappropriate. Given his moderate chronic periodontal disease state, this client requires additional scaling and root planing of active sites, and more aggressive treatment and/or referral for those sites that have not responded to initial treatment. Additionally, his recare interval for treatment should be 3 to 4 months.

18. **A** This client's hypertensive medications may contribute to excessive bleeding during scaling. To avoid excessive bleeding, treatment should be limited to a small area at each visit. Therefore, scaling one quadrant per visit is recommended. Additionally, history of stroke may also be taken into consideration to limit procedures done at each appointment.

19. **B** The clinical photographs of this client reveal intact papilla. The use of interdental brushes for cleaning interproximally would not be indicated. This client's arthritis and self-reported difficulty using floss would be indicators for the use of an automatic toothbrush and floss-holding devices. Use of fluoride mouth rinse is a simple, safe, and cost-effective method of increasing caries protection for an aging population. In addition to this client's generalized recession, which increases his risk of root caries, xerostomia associated with antihypertensive medications further enhances caries development indicating the need for home fluoride use. Oral irrigation devices may be useful

for the furcation areas and deep pockets that have not responded to treatment.

20. **D** The margination of an interproximal overhang can best be accomplished with the use of a fine fluted carbide bur because it fits into the proximal space, adapts to the tooth, and removes the amalgam without much damage to the tooth structure. Diamond finishing strips are difficult to use in the posterior regions of the mouth and are best suited for composite and glass ionomer restorative margination. A gold knife is better suited for the removal of a composite restorative flange. The flame-shaped diamond will not adapt to the tooth surface adequately.

CASE F

1. **E** Because the bone loss on the mesial aspect of the mandibular left second premolar is horizontal, the pocket is suprabony. An infrabony pocket is associated with vertical bone loss. A gingival or pseudopocket is not associated with bone loss. There is no such entity as a mucogingival pocket.

2. **D** American Academy of Periodontology case type Class IV is the correct response. The client's average pocket depth is between 5 and 6 mm and there is moderate bone loss observable on the radiographs. There is bone loss in furcation areas of multirooted teeth and greater than 50% bone loss in the mandibular anterior region. These observations indicate Class IV case type for this client.

3. **C** In the 1950s, Glickman developed the classification of furcation involvement identified by Grades I through IV. In Grade III furcations the bone is not attached to the dome of the furcation. Grade III is characterized by the absence of interradicular bone visible radiographically with the entrance to the furcation occluded by the gingiva.

4. **C** Chronic atrophic candidiasis is also known as denture stomatitis and is limited to the mucosa covered by a full or partial denture. Torus palatinus is an overgrowth of bone and exhibits as a raised surface and a paler diffuse color than the surrounding area. Melanin pigmentation most commonly presents in dark-skinned individuals and appears as a blue, black, or brown color. Primary herpetic gingivostomatitis presents as vesicles in the mouth and is painful. While herpetiform apthous ulcers are tiny in appearance, they are painful, which is not a complaint of this client.

5. **D** The *genial tubercles* are seen as a radiopacity on this mandibular incisor periapical radiograph. A *retrocuspid papilla* is a gingival landmark seen clinically on the lingual gingiva of mandibular canines and is not detectable radiographically. The *symphysis* is a bony landmark located along the border of the mandible and is not evident in this projection. The *mental foramen* is a radiolucent circle often observed on mandibular premolar projections. *Trabeculae* are radiopaque areas of bone that gives cortical bone the spongelike appearance and is not the defined circle seen on this film.

6. **B** Heavy calculus deposits throughout the mandibular teeth give the radiopaque appearance seen in this client's radiographs. Because the scalloping continues across the interdental space, this rules out dental

anatomy variations. The clinical appearance rules out this being composite resin. *Cementicles* are microscopic calcifications of the periodontal ligament.

7. **B** The *nasal conchae* or *turbinates* are normal radiographic landmarks that are often observed projecting into the nasal fossa from the more radiopaque lateral walls of the nasal cavity The conchae are not calcified and therefore appear less radiopaque than the surrounding bony structures.

8. **D** This radiolucency represents an optical illusion of darkness sandwiched between the more radiopaque bone below and the more radiopaque ledge of heavy calculus above. The radiolucency is further enhanced by the morphology of the tooth root, which presents with an increased concavity further contributing to the optical illusion of radiolucency in this area of the tooth. This optical illusion, called cervical burnout, should not be confused with the radiographic appearance of interproximal caries. Caries, when present, will appear at the contact point between adjacent teeth or just apical to this area and not under the gingival margin at the alveolar crest. Clinically, this tooth does not exhibit wear at the cervical area that would indicate abrasion or abfraction.

9. **E** None of the conditions noted in this question place this client at a greater risk for infective bacterial endocarditis than the general population.

10. **B** Daily brushing of a denture with a denture toothpaste and denture brush is the recommended care to prevent stain accumulation. OTC mouth rinses freshen breath, but do not remove plaque and debris from the denture surfaces. Immersion in sodium hypochlorite (household bleach) or dishwashing detergent is not recommended for acrylic dentures and neither is brushing with a household scouring powder because these products will damage the acrylic denture base and teeth.

11. **D** Due to the client's medical condition of congestive heart failure and difficulty in breathing, a supine position is contraindicated. All of the other procedures should be implemented when communicating with the older adult.

12. **E** The use of epinephrine in oral health care treatment for the client on chronic drug therapy for congestive heart failure should be limited or avoided. Epinephrine constricts the blood vessels that would decrease the antihypertensive effects of most of the prescribed medications for this client.

13. **A** Most clients with a history of congestive heart failure will be on a salt restrictive diet, especially when the underlying cause is hypertension. This client is taking antihypertensive medication that would prohibit the use of a sodium-based agent. Because the client exhibits bone loss and gingival recession, an interdental aid which can adapt to wide embrasures and concave proximal tooth surfaces is indicated. All of these aids are effective for interproximal plaque removal.

14. **A** Due to the client's resumption of smoking a pack of cigarettes daily, tobacco cessation intervention is the most immediate client need, both for the improvement of periodontal status and to eliminate this risk

factor for heart disease. Although oral cancer is an additional risk factor for this client, evidence of a suspicious lesion has not been observed at this time. This client's mastitory function has recently been restored through the fabrication of the maxillary denture, negating the need for implant evaluation at this time. Dietary counseling is more commonly performed for caries control, which this client does not present with. All clients should be treated using universal precautions, as there are no advanced procedures.

15. **C** Clinically and radiographically, the mandibular right central incisor presents with the greatest loss of attachment and bone resorption.

16. **B** Because the calculus on the mandibular anterior teeth is heavy, the best choice of instruments is the universal ultrasonic tip because it is ideal for removal of heavy calculus deposits. A modified ultrasonic tip is not as effective in removal of heavy deposits. A universal curette, an area specific curette scaler or the anterior sickle scaler are appropriate for use on the anterior area, but would not be as efficient as an universal ultrasonic tip.

17. **A** This client's age, smoking habit, and medications will all contribute to a reduced ability for the gingival tissues to heal following scaling. Additionally, the blunted papillary shape will most likely prove difficult to clean further contributing to and increased healing time. Hepatitis C will have no effect on the healing time.

18. **A** If results of initial therapy show improvement then the clinician would expect reductions in bleeding and pocket depth as well as improvement in clinical attachment. Root caries risk, although not a problem for this client to date, may increase following a reduction in gingival inflammation which would now expose a greater portion of the root surface to conditions in the oral cavity. Tooth mobility, particularly in the mandibular anterior region, is a likely outcome of periodontal debridement after the heavy band of calculus is removed. Additionally, debridement of the root surface can cause dentinal hypersensitivity, due to removal of the cementum, which may manifest 3 to 4 days after the procedure.

19. **A** Because of furcation involvement in the posterior teeth and bone loss in the mandibular anterior region, surgical intervention will most likely be required to eliminate pocket depth and restore bone through graft procedures. Pit and fissure sealants and restorative procedures are not indicated based on this client's dentition. Periodontal maintenance is a long-term goal after periodontal stability is achieved. Continued initial therapy is superceded by the need for surgical intervention to achieve health.

20. **D** The denture in the photograph appears to be made of poly methyl methacrylate (MMA) resin acrylic. MMA is the most widely used acrylic in dentistry and is the main component of this denture's base. Bis-GMA acrylics are the main component in composite resins. UEDMA acrylics are polyurethane acrylics used to make athletic mouth protectors and soft, flexible dentures. HEMA and PENTA-P acrylics are placed in dentin bonding agent products.

CASE G

1. **C** The radiographs reveal the presence of implants as the restorative replacement of this client's missing teeth. The implant is surgically placed in the mandible, while the prosthetic, in this case a combination of crowns and pontics bridged together, is considered the superstructure. This superstructure is fixed into place on the implant abutments.

2. **B** A *pontic* refers to the restoration that replaces a missing tooth. In this client, the maxillary left first molar is missing, replaced by a pontic, which is part of a three-unit bridge. The maxillary second premolar and second molar are restored with full crowns. These abutment crowns provide support for the bridge. Veneers are restorations that cover only a portion of the tooth and a cantilever is a pontic crown that is attached to a fixed crown on only one side.

3. **A** G.V. Black established the standard for classifying caries in the early 1900s. This system has since been customarily used for cavity preparations and restorations as well. The mandibular left first molar presents with a Class I restoration, involving the pits and fissures of the tooth. Class II restorations would involve a proximal surface of this posterior tooth, whereas a Class III restoration involves the proximal surfaces of anterior teeth. Class IV restorations involve the incisal angle of anterior teeth and Class V restorations are located on the smooth surface of the tooth near the cementoenamel junction (CEJ).

4. **D** Nonsteroidal anti-inflammatory drugs are reported to cause xerostomia. The other conditions listed are not considered to be adverse reactions directly related to NSAIDs.

5. **C** The left side of the implant consists of a pontic that is considered to be a cantilever pontic. It is possible to restore the area using a pontic that is permanently attached to the fixed bridge on only one side. This restoration is considered sound and should not be suspected of failure.

6. **C** Plasma-sprayed titanium is the current alloy used for osseous implants and as observed on the radiographs, the implant is in the shape of a cylinder, not a screw. Additionally, surgical steel implant screws are no longer used to support fixed restorations, and chromium-cobalt alloy frameworks are used for partial denture frameworks, not implants. Gold alloy pontics may be attached to implants in the oral cavity as a replacement for the missing tooth; tungsten carbide and a blade style are not used for implants in the oral cavity.

7. **A** The radiographs reveal an endosseous implant placed within the bone. Subperiosteal implants are inserted under the periosteum but over the bone, while transosteal implants, also referred to as a mandibular staple, are placed completely through the mandible from under the chin into the oral cavity. Endodontic implants are placed through the root canal of an endodontically treated natural tooth.

8. **B** The pulp of this tooth has produced reparative dentin in response to trauma, probably due to the size and location of the restoration. The pulp chamber of this tooth appears smaller due to the amount of this secondary dentin. This appearance differs radiographically from enamel pearls, which are found between furcations and not within the

pulp chamber. Condensing osteitis is a bony condition and would be observed around the apices of the tooth roots. Hypercementosis would appear as an excess growth of cementum, causing the roots to appear bulbous. An abscess would appear radiolucent on a radiograph.

9. **E** The client's degenerative joint disease was caused by the physical trauma of a car accident. The sequela is pain, which is aggravated by temperature changes and changes in body weight. The dental chair should be adjusted for the least amount of weight being placed on cervical spine C3 to C7 vertebrae. The client should be questioned for feedback to determine the best position.

10. **C** Based upon the clinical and radiographic findings, the depth of the pockets due to calculus and periodontal type, C is the most appropriate dental hygiene care plan. Reevaluation of the pocket depths and bleeding should occur at an interval of 4 to 6 weeks. The traditional prophylaxis is not sufficient time to address the need for nonsurgical periodontal therapy. A gross scale followed by fine scale is only appropriate for acute periodontal diseases. Scheduling four quad scale and root debridement appointments is probably not necessary given this client's periodontal condition.

11. **E** The tufted floss is the one device that would effectively remove plaque from this client's multiple problem areas, i.e., implants, fixed bridge, and open contacts present in this client's oral cavity. Introducing more than one additional device, with specific purposes, will most likely reduce client compliance with self-care recommendations. Therefore recommendation of tufted floss to replace toothpicks will most likely enhance this client compliance. Additionally, tufted floss products have a section of regular floss incorporated for the client's normal interproximal plaque removal needs. Wooden wedges and interproximal brushes address only open embrasures. Powered flossing devices are beneficial for those clients who do not floss at all, whereas this client has already developed flossing skills. The end-tuft brush is a toothbrush for specialized brushing needs and this client needs an improved interproximal cleaning method.

12. **A** Implants can be easily scratched by metallic instruments so instruments selected for use should be softer than the implant material. Instruments made of plastic, graphite, or those that are gold-plated or made of nylon are indicated for implants.

13. **B** The best explanation for the localized lack of tissue response is that bacteria from the carious lesion observed radiographically on the distal of the mandibular left premolar may be causing continuous reinfection (seeding) of the gingiva in the adjacent area. A 1-month evaluation is an appropriate interval in which to observe tissue healing following treatment. In fact, a generalized improved tissue condition is noted. Past radiation exposure incurred from medical radiographs would not affect tissue healing and undetected systemic conditions that may influence gingival health would most likely have a generalized manifestation.

14. **E** This client reports having implants for 3 years. Initially, oral hygiene instruction on implant care should be monitored weekly until the client can control plaque accumulation. It is recommended that periodontal

maintenance appointments be scheduled for 1 to 2 month intervals for the first year after surgery. A personalized appointment plan is followed subsequently based on evaluation of implant success, tissue response, and client compliance with self-care recommendations.

15. **D** The best indicator of implant success is mobility (indicating lack of osseointegration), therefore, radiographic examinations along with mobility tests are the most reliable assessment measures. Diseased tissue may not reveal changes in color or gingival contour. Bleeding may be related to probing force and wounding of the tissue, and therefore is not the ideal indicator of healthy or diseased peri-implant tissue.

16. **B** For light calculus and shallow pocket depths, the universal curet can be used for all supra- and subgingival deposits. Root exposure appears to be minimal considering the shallow pocket depths. The area-specific Gracey curets would require frequent and time-consuming instrument transfers. Sickle scalers and the periodontal file should be avoided where root instrumentation would risk gouging with straight cutting edges or a sickle scaler's pointed toe. Graphite instruments would be selected for use in the anterior region, which presents with a dental implant.

17. **C** The use of 0.12% chlorhexidine gluconate rinse is indicated following professional instrumentation when peri-implantitis is present. This client has an increased risk of dental caries as evidenced by the carious lesion present on the distal surface of the mandibular left second premolar as well as root exposure and subgingival plaque. The use of chlorhexidine to prevent caries by combating the elevated levels of streptococcus mutans and lactobacelli, is well supported in the literature. If fluoride was indicated, the best agent to prevent root caries would be water fluoridation versus stannous fluoride toothpaste or low-potency over-the-counter fluoride rinses. Based on the age of this client and the condition of his remaining unrestored teeth (the premolars), pit and fissure sealants would not be significantly beneficial. Potassium oxalate is an ingredient in desensitizing agents and does not appear to be indicated for use by this client.

18. **B** Acidic fluoride may corrode titanium implants; therefore only neutral sodium fluoride at low concentrations should be recommended. While the other preventive procedures listed may not be recommended at this time, based on all client assessment data, there is no contraindication for their use.

19. **C** Calcium sulfate alpha-hemihydrate describes the manufactured product, dental stone, used to construct this client's diagnostic casts. Calcium sulfate dihydrate is the naturally occurring form of gypsum and calcium sulfate hemihydrate and does not adequately describe dental stone. Calcium sulfate beta-hemihydrate is the calcium powder product, plaster of Paris.

20. **E** The maxillary base cut was excessive, giving the diagnostic cast a thin base on the right side. All tooth structures are present. The occlusal plane is parallel to the base and there is one half inch or less of stone base. The mandibular second molar is missing in this client's mouth and was not fractured off the cast during trimming.

CASE H

1. **A** Nicotine stomatitis is characterized by red raised dots at the openings of minor salivary gland ducts on the hard palate. Cigarette smoking is associated with these lesions that should be distinguished from these other conditions. Although burn trauma from hot foods may appear similar, this client's history of tobacco use should be taken into consideration. Hyperkeratosis presents as white lesions on any surface of the oral mucosa. Pyogenic granuloma presents as a single red lesion on the oral mucosa. Kaposi's sarcoma is purplish in color and is found on the hard palate or gingiva.

2. **E** The alveolar mucosa lines the inner surface of the lips and cheeks. This tissue is not attached to the underlining structures and vessels located beneath make this area appear redder in color than the nearby masticatory mucosa. The alveolar mucosa is differentiated from the paler pink attached gingiva by the mucogingival line. The free or marginal gingiva appears as the gingival crest nearest the incisal edge of the tooth and is covered by the oral epithelium. The junctional epithelium is not visible clinically as it is located at the base of the sulcus.

3. **D** Two important public health issues in the United States are the the use of tobacco and the abuse of alcohol. They cause more medical and social problems than all other drugs combined. Additionally, numerous studies provide strong evidence for the relationship between smoking and drinking and the development of squamous cell carcinoma.

4. **D** This client reports a use of OTC medications to alleviate his stomach pain. While his use of these products is frequent, it is in response to stomach irritation caused by excessive alcohol use and not as a result of alcohol-induced craving. Each of the other conditions (hand tremors, rapid pulse rate, xerostomia, and swollen parotid glands) are indicative of a heavy alcohol user.

5. **A** Chronic alcohol use frequently causes benign bilateral parotid swellings called sialadenosis. The parotid gland becomes enlarged and soft. Reduced salivary output (xerostomia) allows for the overgrowth of oral microorganisms and acute caries. However, caries does not spread from tooth to tooth. Carious lesions begin within the enamel and progress into the tooth tissue.

6. **A** This radiolucency is most likely a periapical abscess. The large carious lesions evident on this tooth are most likely the cause of the pulpal necrosis and the resultant inflammatory lesion that appears as a radiolucency at the apex of the affected tooth. When the inflammation becomes chronic, granulation tissue begins to infiltrate the lesion and entrapped epithelial tissue may result in the formation of an apical cyst. While it is difficult to distinguish between a periapical abscess and cyst radiographically, the term *residual cyst* would not be applied here since the affected tooth is present. A residual cyst is left intact when the affected tooth is extracted. If this radiolucency had been a normal anatomic landmark, such as the lingual foramen, it would appear separated from the tooth by the appearance of an intact lamina dura. Additionally, the lingual foramen usually appears radiographically encircled by the radiopaque genial tubercles. Condensing osteitis appears as radiopaque.

7. **D** The mandibular left central incisor appears sound both clinically and radiographically. The maxillary right lateral and central incisors and the maxillary left lateral incisor all appear carious clinically and the radiographs reveal irregular radiolucencies of the mesial and distal surfaces. The mandibular right lateral incisor presents with composite restorations, which appear defective on the mesio-incisal surface.

8. **A** Non-alcohol-containing preprocedural mouth rinses are recommended for the alcoholic client and the client with xerostomia.

9. **A** Oral signs and symptoms of folic acid deficiency include red, sore, swollen, and burning tongue; angular cheilosis; and gingivitis. Multiple vitamins, organ meats, and green vegetables all contain folic acid; however, due to the client's deficiency, a 1 mg supplement three times a week is recommended.

10. **C** While it is true the client is underweight, the dental hygienist would be beyond his or her scope of practice to counsel him for weight gain. The xerostomia induced loss of taste can be treated by use of salivary substitutes. It is within the dental hygienist's scope of practice to counsel the client for xerostomia and its effects on the oral cavity.

11. **A** Because the patient has decision-making capacity, he is then able to give informed consent. Decision-making capacity is the standard that varies with the level of risk to the client. Since scaling and root debridement has a low level of risk as compared to a high level of risk such as cancer treatment, the client's level of understanding and reasoning is adequate. It is in the client's best interest to have the scaling performed and the dental hygienist is not using the right of therapeutic privilege since this is not an emergency procedure in which the client cannot give informed consent. Therefore, the dental hygienist should treat the client.

12. **B** The saliva contains peroxidases, lysozymes, and specific antibodies that have anticariogenic properties. A deficiency of saliva allows for the overgrowth of bacteria and caries development. While poor oral hygiene and consumption of famotidine in chewable mint form are contributing factors, the sequela of xerostomia is the acute caries process.

13. **B** While this client could benefit from all of these procedures, the dental caries process would best be treated with salivary substitutes and stimulants. Xerostomia creates an environment for multiple caries. Correcting the saliva flow will improve the oral balance to reduce subsequent caries formation.

14. **B** Because this client exhibits signs of recent alcohol consumption and based on his reported lifestyle, alcohol withdrawal syndrome may manifest during the oral health care treatment appointment. Alcohol withdrawal may occur within a few hours after the last drink. In fact, he already exhibits hand tremors, nervousness, and a rapid pulse rate, which are all indicative of alcohol withdrawal syndrome.

15. **C** Keeping scheduled appointments is one of the major problems of the alcohol abuser. Because this client's lifestyle revolves around drinking this becomes a priority for him. The difficulty for the alcohol abuser comes from having to make appointments ahead of time. Because drinking and drinking lifestyles take priority he cannot guarantee that he will

be able to keep a scheduled appointment on any given day in the future. While he appears nervous, fear regarding dental treatment has probably not been the primary reason behind his broken appointments. This client reports that the appearance of his teeth may be preventing him from securing better disc jockey jobs, which indicates his interest in achieving appropriate knowledge regarding the care of his oral health.

16. **D** Due to the advanced state of dental caries, the maxillary left central and lateral incisors are not the best choice for a stable finger rest. These teeth may fracture with the applied pressure. The maxillary left canine/premolar area is the best location to attain the most leverage during instrumentation. Using the palm of the hand to fulcrum on the client's chin is an accepted extraoral fulcrum for the maxillary left posterior facial aspects (although of last resort). Fulcruming on the same tooth being instrumented may seem to be considered acceptable. However, it carries a high risk of percutaneous exposure from instrument slippage.

17. **B** The etiotropic phase, or phase I therapy consists of procedures that are designed to control or eliminate the etiologic factors of the disease process. Education and plaque control instruction occur at the beginning of this phase followed by scaling and root debridement. The purpose of the preliminary phase is to bring critical situations under control such as this client's periapical abscess. Phase III, or surgical phase involves regenerative techniques to help restore periodontal tissues that have been lost due to disease. Therapy usually involves restoration and replacement of lost teeth. This client will then remain in the maintenance phase for a lifetime to continuously monitor his periodontal health.

18. **C** This client's teeth would benefit from cosmetic treatment procedures. Additionally, he has expressed a desire to improve his appearance. However, due to the extensive carious lesions, tooth-colored restorative material such as composites will significantly improve his appearance. Furthermore, tooth whitening is contraindicated for individuals with a history of stomach ulcers. Swallowing the bleaching material substance in trays can pose a health risk to the client.

19. **E** This client's self-treatment of his stomach pain with OTC antacids should be investigated by a physician. He should be referred for a physical examination. This client should be educated as to the role nutrition, alcohol consumption, and cigarette smoking play in oral health as well as general health. The dental hygienist should help motivate the client to take responsibility for his oral health through appropriate health behavior and help him understand the importance of regular oral hygiene care.

20. **C** This client's dental conditions are considered chronic and he is not in pain. While his oral exam indicates that he is in need of extensive dental treatment, his lack of a diagnosis concerning his stomach pain, and his unchecked excessive alcohol consumption make extensive, invasive dental treatment risky at this time. He currently exhibits alcohol withdrawal symptoms, which could escalate into confusion and distortion affecting his decision-making regarding consent to dental treatment. Additionally, elevated blood pressure and seizures may result as

alcohol withdrawal syndrome progresses. A physician's examination may indicate that this client should be referred for medication, counseling, and or psychiatric intervention during modification of his alcohol use. Once a medical examination has been done and his physical condition is stabilized, referral should be made to address his nutritional status. Additionally, counseling in smoking cessation and recovery groups such as Alcoholics Anonymous (AA) can be recommended.

CASE I

1. **A** Gingival enlargement is a known side effect of the drug phenytoin. This enlargement, or hyperplasia, in turn, makes plaque control difficult, resulting in gingival inflammation that may further contribute to enlargement of the gingiva.

2. **D** Bacterial plaque accumulation at the gingival margin for over 10 days will result in gingival inflammation. The initial flora of gram-positive cocci and rods and gram-negative cocci give way to an increase in anaerobic and gram-negative motile rods and spirochetes. When these bacteria accumulate in high concentrations as a result of poor home care, the result is gingival inflammation.

3. **D** The Plaque Index of Silness and Loe measures the amount of plaque at the gingival margin. A score of 0 indicates that the tooth is plaque-free. A score of 1 indicates slight plaque, only detectable by swiping a probe across the tooth. A score of 2 indicates that plaque accumulation is observable with the naked eye as a thin film and a score of 3 indicates heavy accumulation.

4. **C** This client's medications produce dryness in the oral cavity. Combined with mouth breathing, the habitually parted lips have become thickened and cracked. Lips of persons with mental retardation are often larger than those found in non-retarded persons, hence this client has developed the habit of licking his lips, which keeps them constantly bathed in saliva. Evaporating moisture adds to the drying effect. Although a person with seizure disorder may accidentally bite the lips during convulsions, the appearance of this client's lips do not indicate a traumatic injury.

5. **C** Because this finding is noted to be hard upon palpation, and no signs of pathosis are present on the radiographs, a bony exostosis is concluded.

6. **E** The paired parallel radiopaque lines outlining this radiolucency indicate the presence of the mandibular canal, which appears to traverse the body of the mandible. This is the normal appearance of this anatomic landmark and should not be mistaken for a bone fracture. Additionally, this landmark should not be confused with the appearance of a nutrient canal. Nutrient canals appear as thin radiolucent lines, usually running in a vertical position when observed in a radiograph of the mandible. While the internal oblique ridge and mylohyoid line may be imaged in this region of the mandible, the density of these anatomic structures makes them appear radiopaque.

7. **B** The radiographic artifact seen on the maxillary left molar periapical radiograph is the result of static electricity. Static electricity creates a lightning bolt-like line of radiolucency on the film. This artifact should not be confused with a torn emulsion or fingernail marks that will appear as white marks on film in the area where the emulsion is missing. Other radiolucent artifacts such as roller marks will appear as uniform radiolucencies seen in a horizontal or vertical position on the film. Fixer contamination would appear radiopaque.

8. **D** The radiographs reveal supernumerary teeth (fourth molars) in the third molar region. The image of a tooth, including the enamel, dentin, and pulp chambers can be identified in these radiographs.

9. **E** Although this client's medications have controlled his seizure episodes for the past 8 months, his medical history indicates that the dental hygienist should prepare for the incidence of a generalized tonic-clonic convulsion. To help minimize the risk of an episode, appointments should be made within a few hours of taking the medications designed to control them. Additionally, the dental hygienist should question the client about any known precipitating factors and ask the client to report the aura sensation. Appropriate actions, such as removing dental instruments from the oral cavity and lowering the dental chair to a supine position, can be performed by the dental hygienist in the event of a seizure. The client should be allowed to rouse on his own from the deep sleep that normally follows the seizure. Seizures usually last no longer than 5 minutes. During this time the client should be monitored for respiratory difficulty as it may be necessary to administer oxygen. Performing CPR is not usually required action during or following the seizure.

10. **C** Because this client's epileptic seizures are exacerbated by loud noises, it may be prudent to forego the use of an ultrasonic scaler. With his heavy plaque and gingival pocketing, all the other listed procedures are acceptable.

11. **C** This client's chief concern is that he has lost his toothbrush. His concern indicates that he knows taking care of his oral health is important for good health. His probable response to oral healthcare instructions will be that he has not been able to perform adequate oral healthcare because of his stolen toothbrush. The best approach to home care instruction is to provide him with a new toothbrush. Providing a toothbrush with his name on it will further motivate this client by addressing his chief concern.

12. **B** The side effects of anticonvulsant drugs may include increased incidence of postscaling gingival bleeding and delayed healing time. This client is taking multiple drugs with this side effect. Given the severity of the gingival inflammation and the spontaneous gingival bleeding that this client presents with, a pretreatment bleeding time would be prudent prior to subgingival instrumentation, including irrigation. Furthermore, the use of anticonvulsants contraindicates the use of NSAIDs and alcohol-containing mouth rinses. Many anticonvulsants can decrease platelet aggregation, which can be exacerbated by the use of NSAIDs. Xerostomia, a side effect of many anticonvulsant drugs, will be exacerbated by the use of alcoholic products. This client's medical history does not indicate the need for premedication.

13. **A** This client has decision-making capacity because he can make a decision independently. Decision-making capacity is not based on overall intelligence. The client need only to be able to understand information and be aware of his well-being.

14. **D** This client's odontogenic infection is located around his impacted mandibular third molars and involves many species of gram positive and gram negative microorganisms. *Streptococcus mutans,* while a primary cause of dental caries, is not seen in odontogenic infections.

15. **D** The photographs reveal a partially supragingival calculus deposit. This deposit must be removed by using a universal curet.

16. **D** Saline irrigation is the first course of treatment for this client. At this time the dentist can prescribe antibiotics for use immediately preceding oral surgery. Cleaning under the operculum with a scaler is contraindicated as is the use of doxycycline.

17. **A** Anticonvulsants taken by this client are partly responsible for his gingival enlargement. While meticulous home care will likely reduce the gingival inflammation caused by the accumulation of bacterial plaque at the gingival margin, the fibrotic enlargement caused by the anticonvulsants will probably remain.

18. **A** Drug interaction between carbamazepine and doxyclycline reduces doxycycline effect. Postscaling pocket treatment could include the use of a stannous fluoride or povidone-iodine irrigation or saline rinse of the posterior pockets instead.

19. **B** Given his medical history, uncontrolled muscle motor movements in this client indicate the onset of an epileptic seizure. The client should be placed in a supine position, on his side to avoid aspiration and respiratory difficulties. Monitor vital signs that indicate the need for supplemental oxygen support. The client's head and other body parts should be protected from trauma by passive restraint. The client should not be forcibly restrained, but care should be taken to prevent contact with objects in the area that may cause injury.

20. **C** Due to the isolated nature of this periodontal condition and the need for anesthesia for the first premolar, the middle superior alveolar injection is indicated.

CASE J

1. **C** While many medications can cause xerostomia, this is not the case for this client. Polyuria is the increased volume of urine in the diabetic client. The blood glucose level prevents the kidneys from reabsorbing water causing dehydration and subsequent xerostomia.

2. **A** The client's medical history indicates that she has type 1 diabetes which results from β-cell destruction by the immune system usually leading to complete absence of insulin production. Although usually arising in puberty, type 1 diabetes may occur at any age. Type 2 diabetes involves insulin resistance with abnormal secretion of insulin, which is not the case in this client. This client is receiving human insulin because of her complete lack of insulin production and is not based on a resistance of the cells to be able to utilize the insulin

produced by the body. Insulin-dependent diabetes mellitus (IDDM), non-insulin-dependent diabetes mellitus (NIDDM), and juvenile diabetes are former names that described the pharmacologic management and age of onset of diabetic clients. These terms were replaced with the etiology-specific type 1 and type 2 classifications.

3. **C** Because this client developed diabetes at the age of 9, does not secrete any insulin herself, and must take several shots each day, it is evident that she has type 1 diabetes. In type 1 diabetes, the immune system produces antibodies against the normal cell components, which attack these molecules, and in the process rapidly destroys this insulin-producing β-cell. Insulin resistance and inadequate insulin secretion are the causes of type 2 diabetes. The pancreas produces insulin, but is unable to use it. Hyperglycemia with ketoacidosis is not the etiologic factor (cause) of type 1 diabetes, but is the result of hypoinsulinism (relative or absolute lack of insulin). About 80% of people with type 2 diabetes are overweight, which may influence insulin resistance. Sucrose consumption is not a cause of diabetes.

4. **B** Dental dysplasia is unrelated to poor glycemic control. However, this client may have an increased risk of experiencing all of the other listed conditions. The risk of dental caries increases as a result of increased glucose in parotid saliva during uncontrolled periods. Additionally, hyperglycemia increases pulse rate and lowers blood pressure. Weight loss in diabetics is the result of uncontrolled hyperglycemia. Due to the inability to use the glucose (due to a lack of insulin), body fat stores are metabolized resulting in weight loss.

5. **B** G. V. Black established the standard for classifying dental caries in the early 1900s. According to this system, the maxillary left first molar presents with a Class II lesion. Class II indicates caries present on the occlusal or facial or lingual surfaces of premolars and molars or the lingual surface of maxillary incisors and proximal surface of the tooth. This lesion can be detected visually (occlusal surface) and radiographically (distal surface). Class I restorations would involve a proximal surface of this posterior tooth, whereas a Class III restoration involves the proximal surfaces of anterior teeth. Class IV restorations involve the incisal angle of anterior teeth and Class V restorations are located on the smooth surface of the tooth near the cementoenamel junction (CEJ).

6. **A** In a Class I occlusal relationship the mesiobuccal cusp of the maxillary first permanent molar occludes with the buccal groove of the mandibular first permanent molar. On the other hand, the buccal groove of the permanent mandibular first molar is distal to the mesiobuccal cusp of the permanent maxillary first molar in a Class II occlusal relationship and mesial in a Class III occlusal relationship. The two divisions of Class II occlusal relationship refer to the maxillary anterior teeth positions. In a Class II–Division 1 occlusal relationship, the mandible is retruded and all of the maxillary incisors are protruded. One or more of the maxillary incisors is in a retruded position in a Class II–Division 2 relationship.

7. **C** The results of self-monitoring of blood glucose levels are the best method to discern control of diabetes. Diabetics will test their blood glucose with a small meter three to four times per day. Good glycemic

control means that the person with diabetes has blood sugar levels (100 to 150 mL/dL) that are close to those of a non-diabetic (80 to 120 mL/dL). Although risk for periodontal disease increases with the duration of diabetes, the duration of diabetes does not effect the control of the disease. Asking the client about adherence to the prescribed schedule of medication, diet, and exercise helps the clinician screen for the risk of dental office emergencies in the client with diabetes. Diabetic emergencies are termed hypoglycemia or ketoacidosis rather than seizure, which is the term used for epileptic convulsive disorders. Diabetics may be at risk for hypertension, however, blood pressure does not indicate level of control of blood glucose in the client with diabetes. Recent unexplained weight loss may be a sign of the onset of type 1 diabetes but the client's weight alone is not indicative of onset of type 1 diabetes.

8. **E** Oral hypoglycemic agents are used to treat clients with type 2 diabetes but not type 1 diabetes as exhibited by this client. All clients with type 1 diabetes require exogenous insulin for survival. Approximately 40% of type 2 diabetics use injected insulin in conjunction with oral hypoglycemic agents, diet, and exercise.

9. **A** An embossed film identification dot is found in one corner of an intraoral radiographic film. This raised bump is used to determine the film's orientation when viewing the radiographic image after processing. During film packet placement intraorally, the embossed dot is positioned at the incisal or occlusal edge of the teeth being imaged. This placement allows the inevitable distortion of radiographic image caused by the bump in the film surface to not interfere with important radiograph interpretation, especially near the tooth apex.

10. **B** A diagnostic-quality periapical radiograph should image the entire tooth from incisal or occlusal edge to the apex plus approximately 2 to 4 mm of supporting bone. Overlapped interproximal spaces would appear as an increased radiopacity as a result of the superimposition of enamel of the adjacent teeth. Cone cutting error presents as a clear or radiopaque error representing an error of no exposure. Herringbone pattern is the name given to the visual pattern of the lead foil imaged onto the film where the film packet is placed in the mouth backward and exposed. Sometimes a film holding device may be imaged onto the resultant radiograph. The radiopacity of this image depends on the material (metal or plastic) of the film holder. However, the radiopacity on this film does not interfere with the diagnostic quality .

11. **A** The midpalatine suture is an opening in the bone that allows more x-rays to pass through to the film, increasing radiolucency. This normal appearance of the midpalatine suture should not be mistaken for a palatal fracture or bone loss. While nutrient canals also appear radiolucent when imaged on a radiograph of the maxillary, they are most often visible as a faint vertical line within the maxillary sinus. The lingual foramen appears as a round radiolucency in the mandibular anterior region.

12. **D** Based on her blood pressure measurement and recent weight loss combined with the tiredness, lethargy, and dry flushed skin, the clinician can conclude that the client is experiencing hyperglycemia with ketoacidosis. The terms hypoglycemia, insulin shock, and insulin

reaction would desinate the clinical findings of normal or slightly elevated blood pressure, anxious, and agitated behavior with moist sweaty skin.

13. **B** Recare appointments scheduled on a regular basis every 3 months is recommended because of the diabetic client's increased susceptibility to periodontal disease.

14. **B** The key factor about the tissue in this region is its color. The gingiva in this region appears red or erythematous.

15. **C** Following tissue injury, first constriction and then dilation of small blood vessels occurs and results in increased blood flow through these vessels. This process is called hyperemia and is responsible for two clinical signs of inflammation: redness (erythema) and heat.

16. **C** Clients with type 1 diabetes have increased susceptibility to periodontal disease evidenced by more frequent and severe duration, more teeth with deep pockets, more alveolar bone loss, and increased tooth mobility.

17. **C** Tissue healing, as demonstrated by an increase in clinical attachment level, is the endpoint of scaling and root debridement. This client presented at her 3-month recare appointment with improved gingival condition due to scaling and root debridement at the initial appointment, which created a root surface conducive to tissue healing.

18. **D** The mandibular first molars and the maxillary right first molar have amalgam restorations on the occlusal surfaces and the dental chart indicates a carious lesion on the maxillary left first molar which contraindicates placement of sealants on these teeth. Additionally the mandibular second molars show signs of sealants and a restoration. The maxillary second molars are well coalesced and show no signs of decay; therefore these teeth would be indicated for sealants.

19. **B** The best preventive agent for this client is home use fluoride. Because diabetics usually suffer from xerostomia and have been shown to have elevated levels of glucose in their parotid saliva they are at increased risk for dental caries. The dental hygienist should assess the best methods for incorporation of fluoride based upon client needs. Diabetics regularly obtain dietary assessment and counseling for their glycemic control. This client's plaque removal is effective as evidenced at her 3-month recare appointment.

20. **C** Fluorosis will not respond well to whitening procedures. While the presence of gingival inflammation as noted in this clients photographs contraindicates whitening procedures that would further irritate the tissue, the inflammation would not affect whitening results. Radiographs reveal no evidence of anterior facial composite restorations and the posterior occlusal sealants will not be an esthetic consideration when considering the use of whitening agents.

The following pages contain the client histories, radiographs, and clinical photographs that are referred to in Cases A–J.

Many of the radiographs and clinical photographs used in the following pages have been cropped, reduced, or enlarged to enhance the clarity of the structures or the lesions they represent.

CLIENT HISTORY SYNOPSIS

Pediatric Client
Maya Patel

VITAL STATISTICS

Age	9	Blood Pressure	100/60 mm Hg
Gender	Female	Pulse Rate	110 bpm
Height	4' 9"	Respiration	20 rpm
Weight	90 lbs.		

1. Under care of physician
   Yes [X]   No [ ]
   Condition: _asthma_

2. Hospitalized within the last 5 years
   Yes [ ]   No [X]
   Reason: _____

3. Has or had the following conditions
   None

4. Current medications
   loratadine (Claritin)—antihistamine
   albuterol (Airet)—adrenergic agonist

5. Smokes or uses tobacco products
   Yes [ ]   No [X]

6. Is pregnant
   Yes [ ]   No [X]   N/A [ ]

MEDICAL HISTORY

This client has had several emergency room visits for breathing difficulty. She is currently under the care of a physician for asthma.

DENTAL HISTORY

This client exhibits an exaggerated gag reflex and mouth breathing. She flosses "sometimes." Impressions for study casts have been indicated to evaluate occlusion.

SOCIAL HISTORY

She lives with both parents and has a younger brother who is 5 years old. Both her parents work outside the home and enjoy a middle-class lifestyle. The family moved to the United States from India 6 years ago and practice the Hindu religion. She is a good student in the fourth grade. Her favorite subject is math and she enjoys poetry.

CHIEF COMPLAINT

She is nervous about dental treatment.

ADULT CLINICAL EXAMINATION

Current oral hygiene status

Generalized marginal plaque accumulation with slight bleeding on probing (BOP).

Supplemental oral examination findings

Upon examination the following were noted:

1. *Slight tongue thrust.*
2. *Maxillary left primary first molar is mobile.*

Clinically visible carious lesion
Clinically missing tooth
Furcation
"Through and through" furcation
Probe 1: Initial probing depth
Probe 2: Probing depth 1 month after scaling and root planing

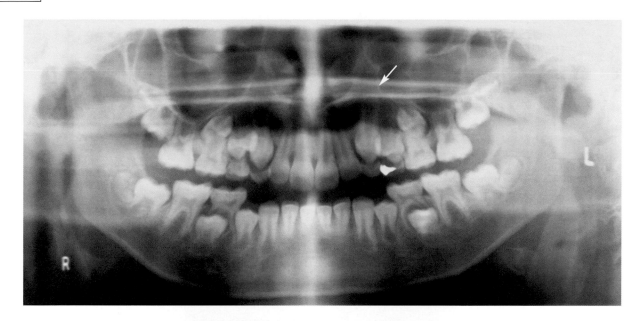

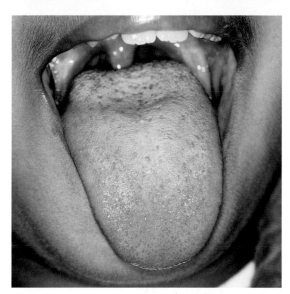

PEDIATRIC CLINICAL EXAMINATION

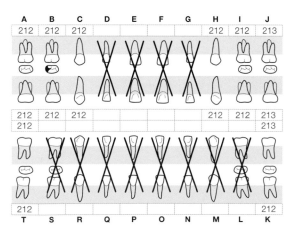

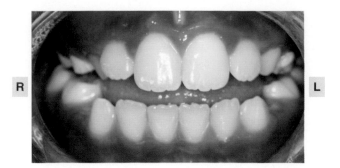

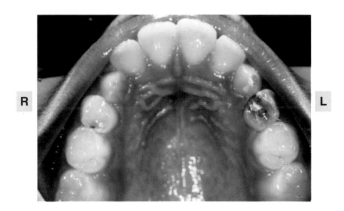

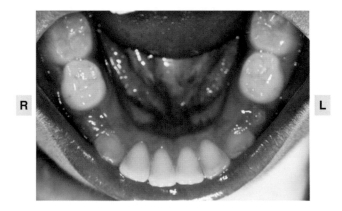

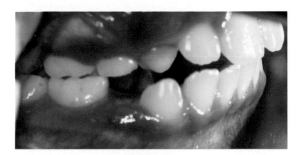

Right side

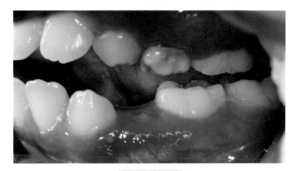

Left side

CLIENT HISTORY SYNOPSIS

Pediatric Client
Zack Ware

VITAL STATISTICS

Age	12	Blood Pressure	110/70 mm Hg
Gender	Male	Pulse Rate	80 bpm
Height	5' 6"	Respiration	18 rpm
Weight	140 lbs.		

1. Under care of physician
Yes ☐ No ☒ Condition: _____

2. Hospitalized within the last 5 years
Yes ☐ No ☒ Reason: _____

3. Has or had the following conditions
none

4. Current medications
none

5. Smokes or uses tobacco products
Yes ☐ No ☒

6. Is pregnant
Yes ☐ No ☐ N/A ☒

MEDICAL HISTORY

This client is in good health.

DENTAL HISTORY

This client grew up in a region with a water supply that contained a high fluoride concentration (greater than 2 ppm). He is currently in maxillary orthodontics and reports that he eats sweets between meals. He breathes through his mouth. His mother reports that he grinds his teeth at night. When asked, he admits to trying spit tobacco.

SOCIAL HISTORY

This client lives with his mother, who works two jobs to make ends meet. He is unsupervised from 3:00 p.m. until 6:00 p.m. Monday through Friday.

CHIEF COMPLAINT

He hates to brush around his braces and the fact that he had to give up his favorite candy while in orthodontic treatment.

ADULT CLINICAL EXAMINATION

	1	2	3	4	5	6	7	8	9	10	11	12	13	14	15	16
Probe 2	X												X			X
Probe 1		323	323	323	312	212	222	323	323	222	223	323		323	323	

	1	2	3	4	5	6	7	8	9	10	11	12	13	14	15	16
Probe 1		323	323	323	323	312	212	212	212	212	213	323		323	323	
Probe 2	X												X			X

R / L

	32	31	30	29	28	27	26	25	24	23	22	21	20	19	18	17
Probe 2	X												X			X
Probe 1		323	323	212	212	212	212	212	212	212	212	212		323	323	

	32	31	30	29	28	27	26	25	24	23	22	21	20	19	18	17
Probe 1		323	323	212	212	212	213	312	212	213	212		323	323	X	
Probe 2	X												X			X

Current oral hygiene status

Generalized marginal plaque accumulation with slight bleeding on probing (BOP).

Supplemental oral examination findings

Upon examination the following was noted:

Mandibular left primary molar is mobile.

⌓ Clinically visible carious lesion
✗ Clinically missing tooth
△ Furcation
▲ "Through and through" furcation
Probe 1: Initial probing depth
Probe 2: Probing depth 1 month after scaling and root planing

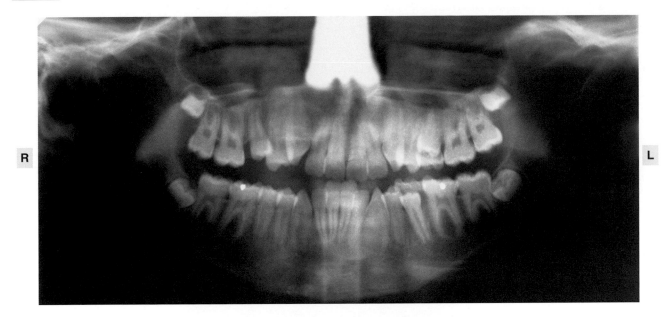

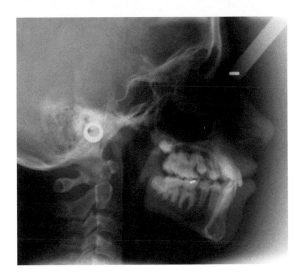

PEDIATRIC CLINICAL EXAMINATION

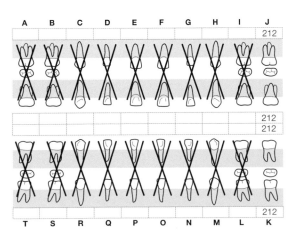

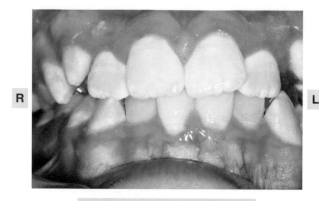

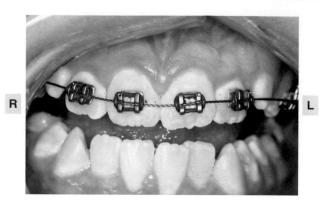

**1 month prior to placement of
orthodontic bands**

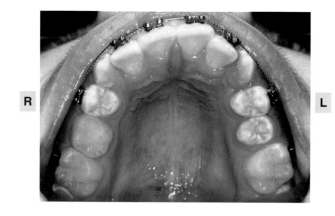

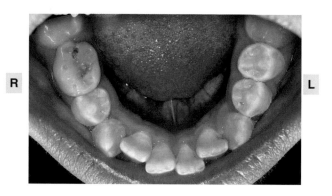

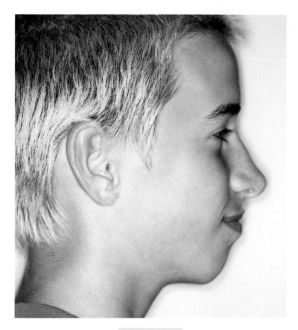

Right side

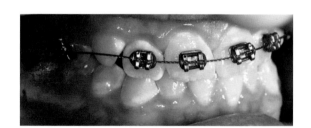

Right side

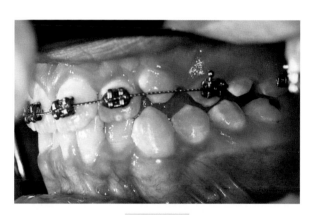

Left side

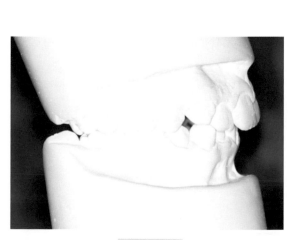

Right side

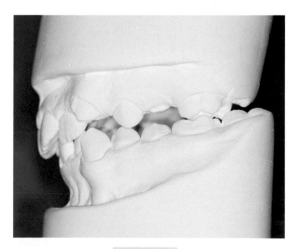

Left side

CLIENT HISTORY SYNOPSIS

Adult Peridontally Involved Client
Katherine Flynn

VITAL STATISTICS

Age	53	Blood Pressure	103/62 mm Hg
Gender	Female	Pulse Rate	72 bpm
Height	5' 2"	Respiration	18 rpm
Weight	105 lbs.		

1. Under care of physician
   Yes [X]   No [ ]
   Condition: angina pectoris,
   rheumatoid arthritis

2. Hospitalized within the last 5 years
   Yes [X]   No [ ]
   Reason: shoulder surgery

3. Has or had the following conditions
   syncope, hormonal replacement therapy,
   tetracycline allergic response

4. Current medications
   acetaminophen (Tylenol)—nonnarcotic analgesic
   diclofenac (Voltran)—nonsteroidal anti-inflammatory
   diltiazem HCl (Cardizem)—calcium channel antagonist, antianginal
   estrogen (Premarin)—hormone replacement

5. Smokes or uses tobacco products
   Yes [ ]   No [X]

6. Is pregnant
   Yes [ ]   No [X]   N/A [ ]

MEDICAL HISTORY

Although not currently taking nitroglycerin, she does keep a prescription for this drug.

DENTAL HISTORY

This client has recently experienced a fainting episode during dental treatment. She reports that her teeth are very sensitive to hot and cold stimulation and that during her last scaling appointment the pain became so intense that she fainted. She was embarrassed by this incident and she appears worried that it will happen today.

This client has been a lifelong resident in a community with optimal levels of fluoride in the water.

SOCIAL HISTORY

This client's husband of 33 years passed away about one and one-half years ago. To help cope with her loss, she re-entered the work force after many years as a homemaker and an active life of volunteerism. Her husband's professional career provided her with financial security, but working at the community college adds more structure to her life since his death. She is determined to "make it on her own."

CHIEF COMPLAINT

This client's chief complaint is the hot and cold sensitivity she experiences, limiting her ability to enjoy certain foods. She is also concerned about the continuing gum recession along her lower anterior teeth.

ADULT CLINICAL EXAMINATION

R / **L**

Maxillary (teeth 1–16):

	1	2	3	4	5	6	7	8	9	10	11	12	13	14	15	16
Probe 2	X	223	X	213	423	212	312	212	222	223	312	323	312	X	X	X
Probe 1	X	112	X	212	313	222	212	212	222	112	312	323	312	X	X	X

	1	2	3	4	5	6	7	8	9	10	11	12	13	14	15	16
Probe 1	X	223	X	324	324	532	333	312	212	212	212	222	223	X	X	X
Probe 2	X	223	X	333	325	532	333	312	212	212	212	323	323	X	X	X

Mandibular (teeth 17–32):

	32	31	30	29	28	27	26	25	24	23	22	21	20	19	18	17
Probe 2	336	822	213	212	212	212	111	111	111	213	311	X	222	X	X	X
Probe 1	337	814	413	313	323	323	111	111	111	212	221	X	111	X	X	X

	32	31	30	29	28	27	26	25	24	23	22	21	20	19	18	17
Probe 1	333	623	423	313	111	321	111	111	123	321	223	X	112	X	X	X
Probe 2	223	723	313	312	122	222	211	112	113	312	313	X	112	X	X	X

Current oral hygiene status

She is meticulous about her home care and she reports "wearing out" her toothbrushes within a "couple of weeks." She uses a scrub method of brushing. Additonally, she uses floss, fluoride rinses, and rubber tip stimulators.

Supplemental oral examination findings

Upon examination the following were noted:

1. *Nocturnal bruxism*
2. *Class I mobility on the mandibular left and right lateral and central incisors and the maxillary left second premolar*

Clinically visible carious lesion

Clinically missing tooth

△ Furcation

▲ "Through and through" furcation

Probe 1: Initial probing depth

Probe 2: Probing depth 6 months after scaling and root planing

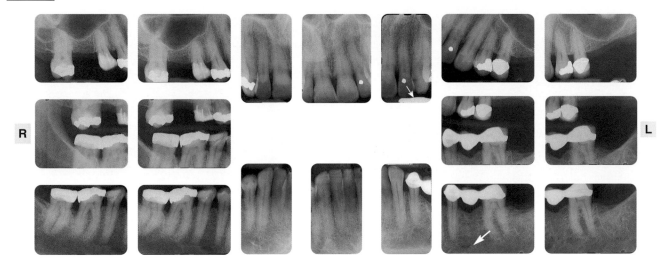

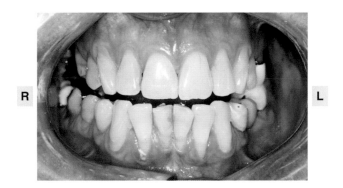

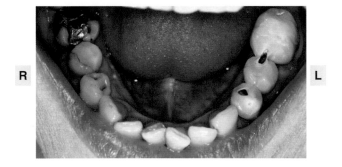

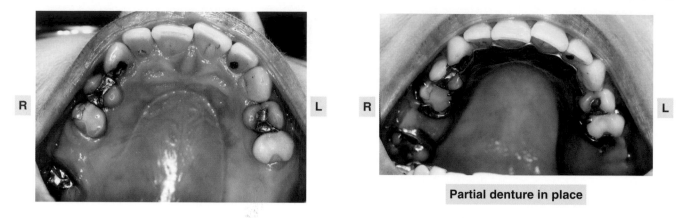

Partial denture in place

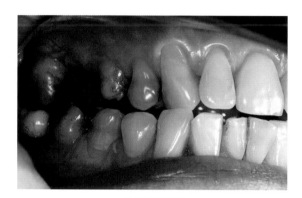

Right side

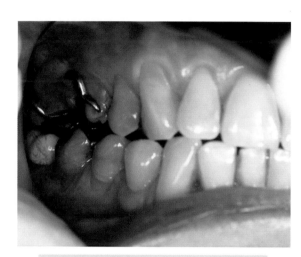

Right side with partial denture in place

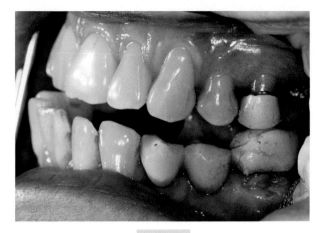

Left side

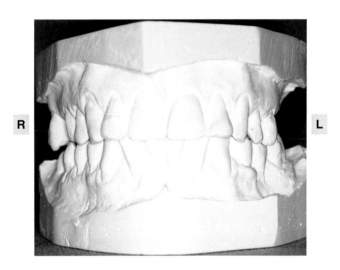

R   L

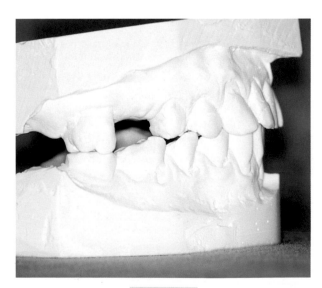

Right side

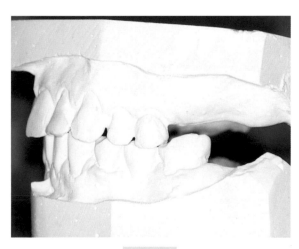

Left side

CLIENT HISTORY SYNOPSIS

Adult Peridontally Involved Client
Louis Riddick

VITAL STATISTICS

Age	56	Blood Pressure	140/90 mm Hg	
Gender	Male	Pulse Rate	70 bpm	
Height	5' 3"	Respiration	17 rpm	
Weight	150 lbs.			

1. Under care of physician
Yes [X] No [ ]
Condition: *blood pressure monitoring*
smoking cessation

2. Hospitalized within the last 5 years
Yes [ ] No [X]
Reason: _____

3. Has or had the following conditions
mild hypertension
_____
_____

4. Current medications
nicotine polacrilex (Nicorette)—smoking deterrent
_____
_____
_____

5. Smokes or uses tobacco products
Yes [ ] No [X]

6. Is pregnant
Yes [ ] No [ ] N/A [X]

MEDICAL HISTORY

This client's hypertension was diagnosed after he attended a blood pressure screening last month. At that time, he received a complete physical exam and was advised to quit smoking. He received advice from his physician to start using a smoking deterrent last week and has not had a cigarette in 5 days.

DENTAL HISTORY

He reports that he had several teeth extracted "years ago," but that he gets along just fine without them. In fact, he jokes, "I now have less to brush."

SOCIAL HISTORY

This client considers his golf outings as exercise and important to his mental well-being. His relationship with his family is important to him and his wife's concern for his dental health is what got him here today.

CHIEF COMPLAINT

He mentioned to his wife last week that his teeth appeared to be getting loose. At first he dismissed this as a natural part of the aging process, until his wife expressed concern. He is here today to find out the cause.

ADULT CLINICAL EXAMINATION

Maxillary (teeth 1–16):

	1	2	3	4	5	6	7	8	9	10	11	12	13	14	15	16
Probe 2 (F)	X	456	859	736	735	423	423	323	323	324	434	533	335	566	X	544
Probe 1 (F)		567	9610	847	846	534	534	434	434	435	545	644	446	677		655
Probe 1 (P)		758	9711	745	446	534	434	434	434	434	335	645	656	757		656
Probe 2 (P)		647	8610	634	335	423	323	323	323	323	224	534	545	646		545

R   L

Mandibular (teeth 32–17):

	32	31	30	29	28	27	26	25	24	23	22	21	20	19	18	17
Probe 2 (L)	444	X	434	433	323	322	222	222	222	323	334	434	X	X	X	555
Probe 1 (L)	655	X	545	544	424	423	222	223	323	324	435	545	X	X	X	666
Probe 1 (F)	655	X	435	534	435	534	323	323	323	324	445	545	X	X	X	656
Probe 2 (F)	544	X	324	423	324	423	323	323	323	223	334	434	X	X	X	545

Current oral hygiene status

Light subgingival plaque especially interproximal was noted and there is generalized bleeding upon probing. He recently began using an automatic toothbrush.

Supplemental oral examination findings

Upon examination the following were noted:

1. *Slight tongue thrust*
2. *Generalized Class I mobility*

Legend:
- Clinically visible carious lesion
- X Clinically missing tooth
- △ Furcation
- ▲ "Through and through" furcation
- Probe 1: Initial probing depth
- Probe 2: Probing depth 1 month after scaling and root planing

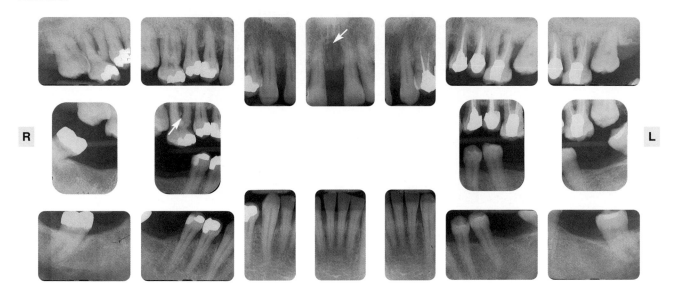

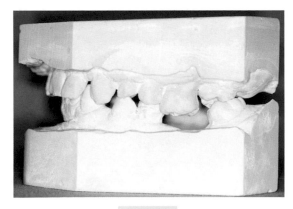

Right side

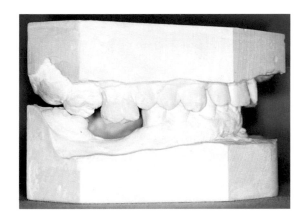

Left side

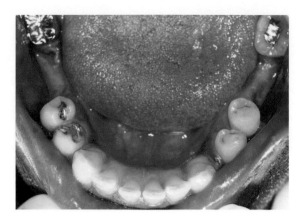

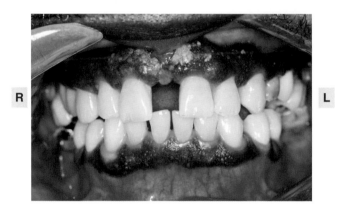

R   L

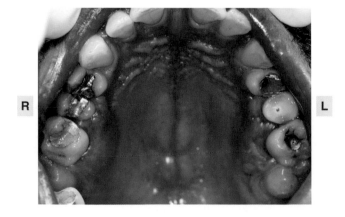

R   L

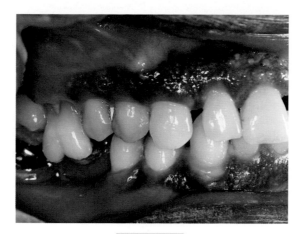

Right side

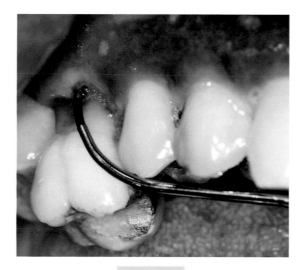

Right side

CLIENT HISTORY SYNOPSIS

Geriatric Client
Juan Hernandez

VITAL STATISTICS

Age	81	Blood Pressure	140/90 mm Hg
Gender	Male	Pulse Rate	70 bpm
Height	5' 10"	Respiration	14 rpm
Weight	175 lbs.		

1. Under care of physician
   Yes [X] No [ ]
   Condition: *hypertension*

2. Hospitalized within the last 5 years
   Yes [X] No [ ]
   Reason: *cerebrovascular accident (CVA)*

3. Has or had the following conditions
   Atherosclerosis, Osteoarthritis

4. Current medications
   aspirin (Bayer)—analgesic/nonsteroidal antiinflammatory drug
   warfarin sodium (Coumadin)—anticoagulant
   chlorthiazide (Diuril)—diuretic
   atvorvastatin calcium (Lipitor)—antihyperlipidemic
   naproxen (Naproxen)—antiinflammatory/antiarthritic

5. Smokes or uses tobacco products
   Yes [ ] No [X]

6. Is pregnant
   Yes [ ] No [ ] N/A [X]

MEDICAL HISTORY

This client reports slightly limited use of his right side since his stroke 5 years ago, and he experiences morning stiffness especially in his hands, hips, and knees.

DENTAL HISTORY

This client is proud that he has all of his teeth and does not wear dentures. He attributes his good oral condition to the "goodness of faith" and the good food of his culture. He brushes once per day and has had instruction in flossing, but his arthritic hands have not "had much luck" using floss.

SOCIAL HISTORY

This client lives with the youngest of his six children. His extended family is close and he enjoys being the family patriarch. His wife of 58 years is deceased.

CHIEF COMPLAINT

This client has noticed that his temporomandibular joint (TMJ) has become somewhat problematic. He noticed an increase in stiffness and a crackling sensation, which has manifested bilaterally.

ADULT CLINICAL EXAMINATION

	1	2	3	4	5	6	7	8	9	10	11	12	13	14	15	16
Probe 2	X	324	425	534	212	212	212	212	212	212	315	434	334	424	434	X
Probe 1	X	324	425	534	212	312	212	212	212	212	315	434	334	434	434	X

	1	2	3	4	5	6	7	8	9	10	11	12	13	14	15	16
Probe 1	X	466	435	523	323	313	212	212	212	212	214	414	424	523	465	X
Probe 2	X	466	435	523	322	212	212	212	212	212	213	314	424	523	444	X

R / **L**

	32	31	30	29	28	27	26	25	24	23	22	21	20	19	18	17
Probe 2	X	525	525	524	414	212	212	212	212	212	214	415	424	424	525	X
Probe 1	X	525	525	524	414	333	322	212	212	212	214	415	525	525	525	X

	32	31	30	29	28	27	26	25	24	23	22	21	20	19	18	17
Probe 1	X	425	526	524	412	212	212	212	212	212	214	412	412	424	433	X
Probe 2	X	424	526	524	412	212	212	212	212	212	214	312	324	423	X

Current oral hygiene status

Bleeding upon probing interproximally in posterior regions is noted. The premolar teeth exhibit fremitus.

Supplemental oral examination findings

Upon examination the following were noted:

1. Moderate xerostomia
2. TMJ moderate crepitus bilaterally
3. Heberden's nodes and Bouchard's nodes on the fingers

- Clinically visible carious lesion
- Clinically missing tooth
- △ Furcation
- ▲ "Through and through" furcation
- Probe 1: Initial probing depth
- Probe 2: Probing depth 1 month after scaling and root planing

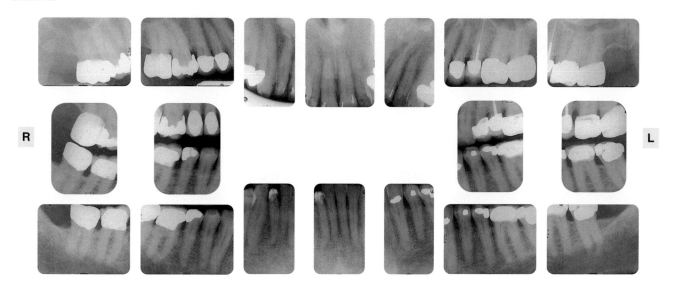

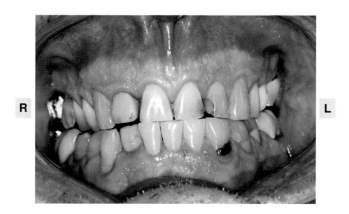

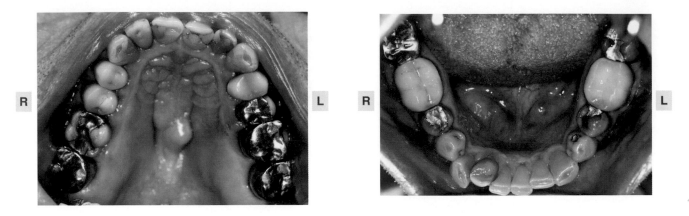

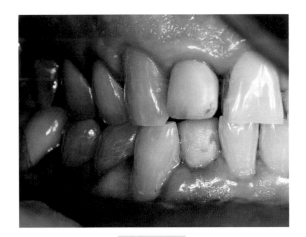

Right side

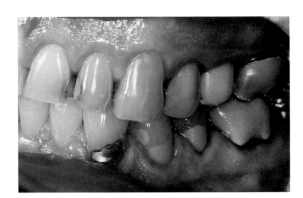

Left side

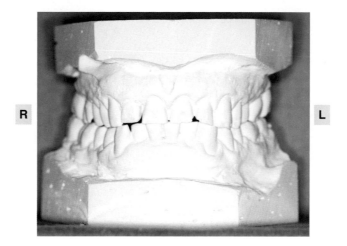

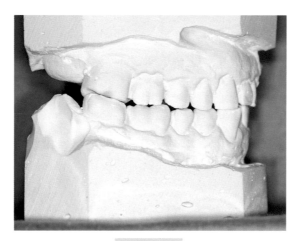

Right side

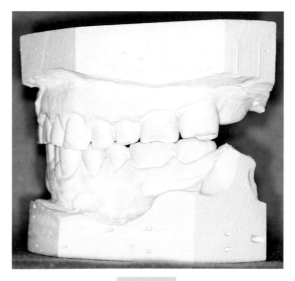

Left side

CLIENT HISTORY SYNOPSIS

Geriatric Client
Virginia Carson

VITAL STATISTICS

Age	66	Blood Pressure	130/100 mm Hg
Gender	Female	Pulse Rate	90 bpm
Height	5' 3"	Respiration	20 rpm
Weight	165 lbs.		

1. Under care of physician
   Yes [X] No [ ] Condition: *congestive heart failure*

2. Hospitalized within the last 5 years
   Yes [X] No [ ] Reason: *heart attack*

3. Has or had the following conditions
   hepatitis C, bronchitis

4. Current medications
   atenolol (Tenormin)—antihypertensive/beta-adrenergic antagonists
   digoxin (Lanoxicaps)—antiarrhythmic/cardiac glycoside
   enalapril maleate (Vasotec)—antihypertensive/angiotension-converting
   enzyme inhibitor
   furosemide (Lasix)—diuretic
   multivitamin with iron (Stress Tabs)—over-the-counter (OTC) dietary supplement

5. Smokes or uses tobacco products
   Yes [X] No [ ]

6. Is pregnant
   Yes [ ] No [X] N/A [ ]

MEDICAL HISTORY

Although her physician has prescribed smoking cessation products, the client has returned to smoking a pack of cigarettes per day.

DENTAL HISTORY

The client has just received a new full maxillary denture last month. Although she has been back to the office several times for adjustments, she appears to be happy with the appliance.

SOCIAL HISTORY

The client is a widow and has lived alone since her husband passed away 9 years ago. Striving to live comfortably on a small pension, the client takes advantage of senior citizen assistance available to her in the community. She recently moved to a senior citizen condominium where she is acquiring a new social life.

CHIEF COMPLAINT

The client's immediate dental complaint has been addressed with regards to her full maxillary denture. Her previous maxillary denture was almost 20 years old. It had chipped teeth and was ill fitting. After fabricating her new denture, she was reffered for dental hygiene comprehensive services. She has made this appointment "out of respect" for the dentist who made her denture. She "promised him" that she would return to the office to "take care of her lower teeth after her denture was made."

ADULT CLINICAL EXAMINATION

Current oral hygiene status

Poor oral hygiene with generalized marginal plaque. She reports that she brushes once a day and has tried flossing, but her teeth are too tight and the floss does not fit between them.

Supplemental oral examination findings

Upon examination the following was noted:

1. Generalized spontaneous gingival bleeding

Maxillary (teeth 1–16): clinically missing teeth.

Mandibular probing depths:

	32	31	30	29	28	27	26	25	24	23	22	21	20	19	18	17
Probe 2		757	555	454	434	534	424	424	424	444	445	555	554	545	635	
Probe 1		757	555	454	434	534	424	434	535	555	555	554	554	545	645	

Maxillary probing depths:

	1	2	3	4	5	6	7	8	9	10	11	12	13	14	15	16
Probe 1		657	635	525	333	434	434	434	434	434	434	434	546	756		
Probe 2		656	635	525	323	333	434	434	434	434	434	434	546	746		

- 🦷 Clinically visible carious lesion
- ✖ Clinically missing tooth
- △ Furcation
- ▲ "Through and through" furcation
- Probe 1: Initial probing depth
- Probe 2: Probing depth 1 month after scaling and root planing

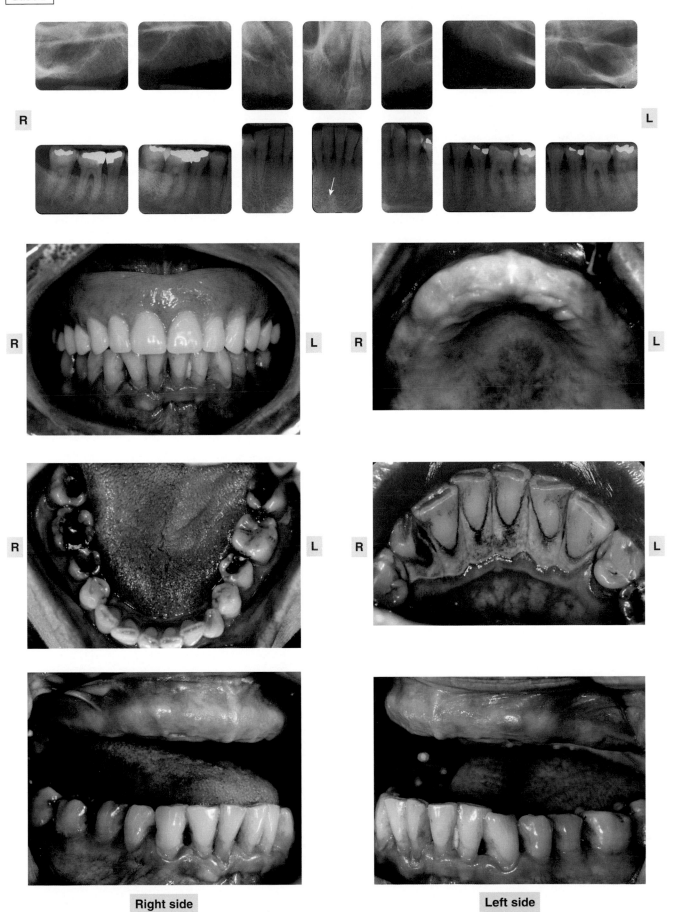

R

L

R   L

R   L

R   L

R   L

R   L

Right side

Left side

CLIENT HISTORY SYNOPSIS

Special Needs Client
Thoroughgood Epps

VITAL STATISTICS

Age	43	Blood Pressure	120/82 mm Hg
Gender	Male	Pulse Rate	63 bpm
Height	6' 0"	Respiration	14 rpm
Weight	190 lbs.		

1. Under care of physician
   Yes [X]   No [ ]
   Condition: osteoarthritis (degenerative joint disease)

2. Hospitalized within the last 5 years
   Yes [X]   No [ ]
   Reason: car accident

3. Has or had the following conditions
   osteoarthritis

4. Current medications
   ketorolac (Toradol)—nonsteroidal antiinflammatory drug

5. Smokes or uses tobacco products
   Yes [ ]   No [X]

6. Is pregnant
   Yes [ ]   No [ ]   N/A [X]

MEDICAL HISTORY

This client is currently being treated for osteoarthritis and reports that his medication helps with the pain, especially in C3–C7 of the cervical spine. He has had numerous x-ray examinations of his neck, back, and chest in the past 3 years.

DENTAL HISTORY

He experienced traumatic injury to his back and mandible following a car accident 3 years ago.

SOCIAL HISTORY

He is single and enjoying a new life since retiring from active military duty.

CHIEF COMPLAINT

Seeking to maintain his oral health since leaving the military.

ADULT CLINICAL EXAMINATION

	1	2	3	4	5	6	7	8	9	10	11	12	13	14	15	16
Probe 2	X	222	313	313	312	212	312	211	212	211	112	112	313	X	323	X
Probe 1		222	225	423	323	313	312	212	212	212	212	212	313		425	
Probe 1		324	413	313	312	222	222	223	312	212	212	223	324		524	
Probe 2		213	213	312	212	211	112	212	212	212	112	112	213		312	

R   L

	32	31	30	29	28	27	26	25	24	23	22	21	20	19	18	17
Probe 2	322	X	223	312	212	212							213	413	X	424
Probe 1	435	X	534	322	322	212							224	334	X	534
Probe 1	435	X	434	423	423	323							334	435	X	534
Probe 2	424	X	324	412	212	213							325	523	X	424

Current oral hygiene status

Light subgingival calculus can be detected interproximally in the posterior regions. Generalized moderate interproximal plaque accumulation was noted with moderate bleeding on probing localized in the maxillary posterior regions. Uses waxed dental floss several times a week and toothpicks after lunch every day. Brushes twice each day using a soft bristle brush in a circular motion; once in the morning and once before going to bed.

Supplemental oral examination findings

None

🦷 Clinically visible carious lesion
✕ Clinically missing tooth
△ Furcation
▲ "Through and through" furcation
Probe 1: Initial probing depth
Probe 2: Probing depth 1 month after scaling and root planing

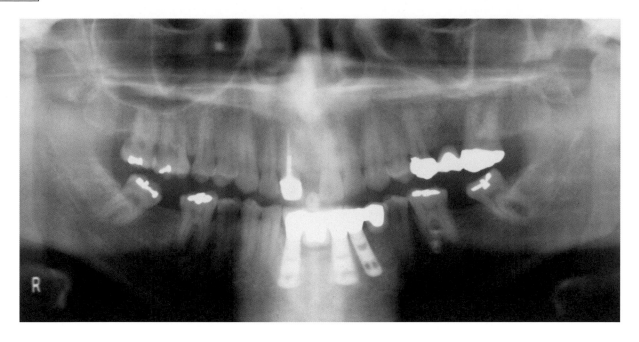

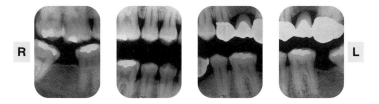

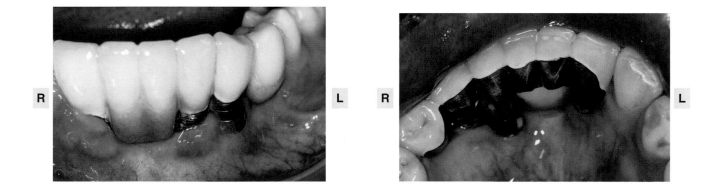

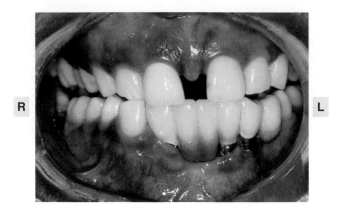

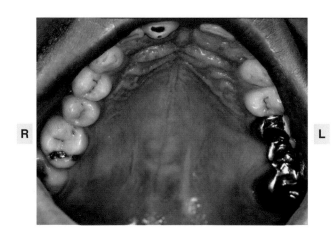

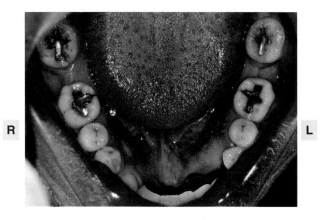

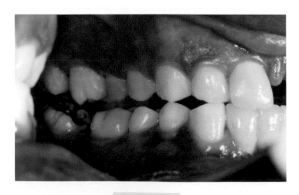

Right side

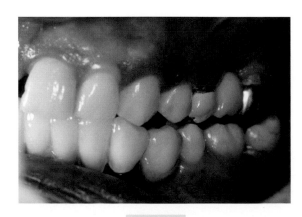

Left side

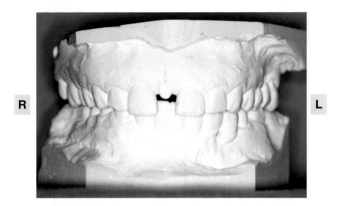

R   L

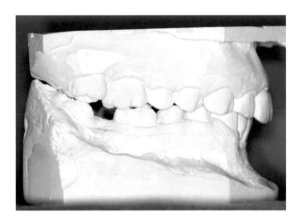

Right side

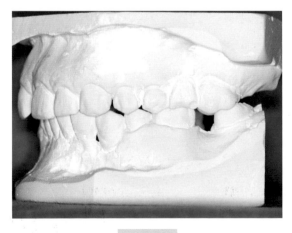

Left side

CLIENT HISTORY SYNOPSIS

Special Needs Client
"Johnnie" Johnson

VITAL STATISTICS

Age	38	Blood Pressure	118/76 mm Hg
Gender	Male	Pulse Rate	90 bpm
Height	5' 10"	Respiration	24 rpm
Weight	160 lbs.		

1. Under care of physician
   Yes ☐ No ☒ Condition: _____

2. Hospitalized within the last 5 years
   Yes ☐ No ☒ Reason: _____

3. Has or had the following conditions
   stomach ulcers
   _____

4. Current medications
   calcium carbonate, magnesium hydroxide (Mylanta)—
   gastrointestinal agent/antacid
   famotidine (Pepcid chewables)—gastrointesinal agent/antacid
   ibuprofen (Advil)—analgesic/nonsteroidal antiinflammatory drug
   magnesium hydroxide, aluminum hydroxide, simethicone (Maalox)—
   gastrointestinal agent/antacid

5. Smokes or uses tobacco products
   Yes ☒ No ☐

6. Is pregnant
   Yes ☐ No ☐ N/A ☒

MEDICAL HISTORY

This client presents with an unremarkable medical history, although anecdotal information may indicate his need for a medical examination. There have been no hospital or medical treatments in his past. He has not had a physical exam in several years and although he is experiencing stomach problems, he has chosen not to see a physician. His current over-the-counter (OTC) medications are self-prescribed.

DENTAL HISTORY

This client has undergone extensive dental restorative work as a child and a teenager, however, he has not received any professional oral health care in the past 10 to 15 years. He has scheduled numerous appointments in the past month, but has either cancelled them or has just not shown up.

SOCIAL HISTORY

This client is somewhat of a "loner." His lifestyle, in which he sleeps during the day and works in nightclubs and after-hours bars at night, prevents him from developing long-term friendships. He states that he often does not know the "real" names of many of the people he encounters. Likewise, "Johnnie" is his working, or stage name, for purposes of his job. His family resides out-of-state and he has not had a permanent residence since moving out of his parents' house. He just recently moved out of a shared apartment to live with his girlfriend in her mobile home.

CHIEF COMPLAINT

This client is not happy with the appearance of his teeth. He reports that he does not have "a lot of money" for dental treatment, however, he has made this appointment at the urging of his new girlfriend. Additionally, he thinks the appearance of his front teeth may be causing him not to get the better DJ opportunities. He aspires to perform disk jockeying services at more upscale dance clubs and parties such as wedding receptions.

ADULT CLINICAL EXAMINATION

	1	2	3	4	5	6	7	8	9	10	11	12	13	14	15	16
Probe 2	535	534	422	323	313	313	313	312	212	213	213	313	323	436	X	636
Probe 1	645	535	544	434	423	323	323	313	313	313	313	423	324	536	X	635
Probe 1	534	424	434	323	313	313	323	323	323	313	323	424	424	434	X	524
Probe 2	433	323	323	313	313	212	213	313	313	313	213	313	423	424	X	424

	32	31	30	29	28	27	26	25	24	23	22	21	20	19	18	17
Probe 2	534	434	433	323	313	313	313	313	313	313	313	313	323	434	X	535
Probe 1	635	534	433	323	323	323	313	313	313	313	413	424	425	535	X	535
Probe 1	535	635	434	423	323	313	423	423	424	324	424	424	435	635	X	536
Probe 2	534	534	423	323	323	212	313	313	313	313	313	313	324	434	X	525

Current oral hygiene status

In spite of this client's lack of professional oral hygiene care over the past several years, his calculus accumlation is slight, however, generalized. He performs oral hygiene self-care reasonably well and consistently. There is slight papillary bleeding on probing.

Supplemental oral examination findings

Upon examination the following were noted:

1. *Slight xerostomia.*
2. *Loss of taste sensation.*
3. *Bilateral parotid gland enlargement.*

⌑ Clinically visible carious lesion

✕ Clinically missing tooth

△ Furcation

▲ "Through and through" furcation

Probe 1: Initial probing depth

Probe 2: Probing depth 1 month after scaling and root planing

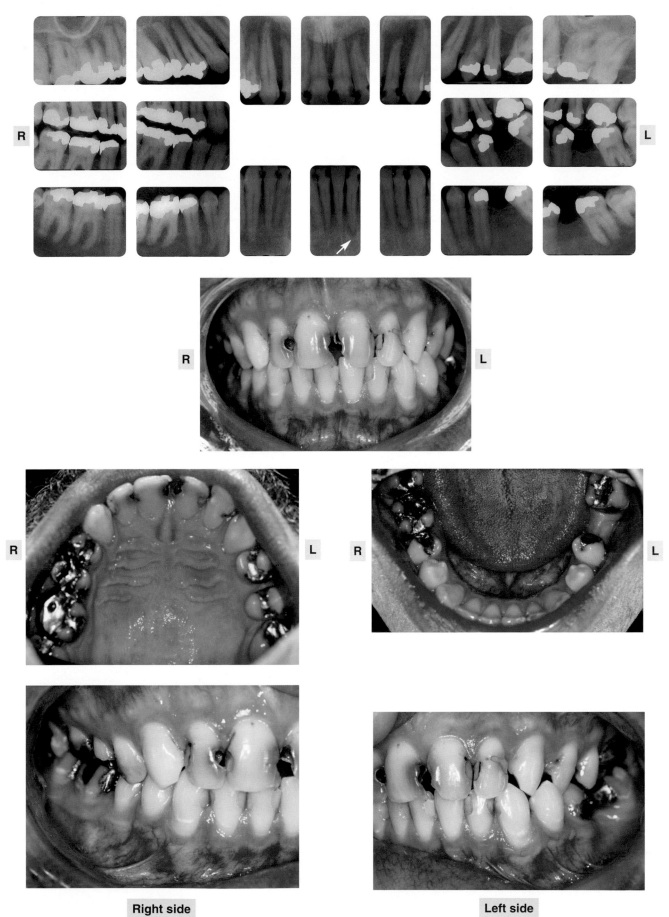

Right side

Left side

CLIENT HISTORY SYNOPSIS

Medically Compromised Client
Thomas Small

VITAL STATISTICS

Age	32	Blood Pressure	135/89 mm Hg
Gender	Male	Pulse Rate	88 bpm
Height	5′ 7″	Respiration	14 rpm
Weight	215 lbs.		

1. Under care of physician
   Yes [X]   No [ ]   Condition: *seizure disorder*

2. Hospitalized within the last 5 years
   Yes [ ]   No [X]   Reason:

3. Has or had the following conditions
   epilepsy

4. Current medications
   carbamazepine (Tegretol)—anticonvulsant
   phenytoin (Dilantin)—anticonvulsant
   topiramate (Topamax)—anticonvulsant
   gabapentin (Neurontin)—anticonvulsant

5. Smokes or uses tobacco products
   Yes [ ]   No [X]

6. Is pregnant
   Yes [ ]   No [ ]   N/A [X]

MEDICAL HISTORY

Thomas Small is mildly retarded. His epileptic seizures are responding well to his current medications and appear to be controlled. His last episode was 8 months ago and his seizures appear to be precipitated by sudden loud noises.

DENTAL HISTORY

This client maintains regular oral healthcare appointments.

SOCIAL HISTORY

This client enjoys his job at the supermarket, and is especially proud that he is learning where items are located in each aisle. He lives in an independent living group home.

CHIEF COMPLAINT

This client thinks one of the other men living at his group home has stolen his toothbrush.

ADULT CLINICAL EXAMINATION

	1	2	3	4	5	6	7	8	9	10	11	12	13	14	15	16
Probe 2																
Probe 1 (F)	844	445	324	314	414	323	323	436	634	434	433	333	333	334	444	444
Probe 1 (P)	878	444	323	323	312	313	212	212	212	212	212	213	313	313	315	888
Probe 2																

	32	31	30	29	28	27	26	25	24	23	22	21	20	19	18	17
Probe 2	X															X
Probe 1 (L)	X	534	323	313	313	424	212	222	222	222	222	223	324	426	428	X
Probe 1 (F)	X	645	433	323	323	324	424	424	424	425	524	223	323	323	456	X
Probe 2	X															X

R — L

Current oral hygiene status

Spontaneous marginal bleeding on probing.

Supplemental oral examination findings

Upon examination the following were noted:

1. *Lips parted in occlusion*
2. *Periocoronitis around mandibular third molars*
3. *Evidence of mouth breathing and excessive lip licking*
4. *Hard nodular projection noted on the maxillary right alveolar ridge*

Clinically visible carious lesion

Clinically missing tooth

△ Furcation

▲ "Through and through" furcation

Probe 1: Initial probing depth

Probe 2: Probing depth 1 month after scaling and root planing

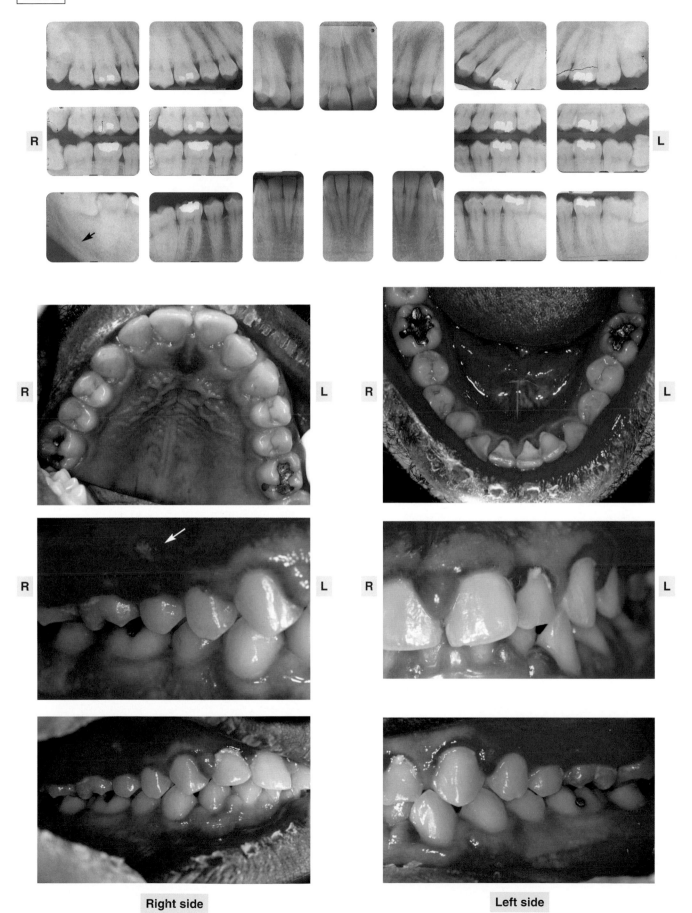

Right side

Left side

CLIENT HISTORY SYNOPSIS

Medically Compromised Client
Nancy Foster

VITAL STATISTICS

Age	21	Blood Pressure	90/60 mm Hg
Gender	Female	Pulse Rate	96 bpm
Height	5' 3"	Respiration	14 rpm
Weight	116 lbs.		

1. Under care of physician
   Yes [X] No [ ]
   Condition: _monitor glycemic control_

2. Hospitalized within the last 5 years
   Yes [ ] No [X]
   Reason: _____

3. Has or had the following conditions
   diabetes

4. Current medications
   regular insulin (Humulin R)
   neutral protein Hagedorn (NPH) insulin suspension (Humulin N)

5. Smokes or uses tobacco products
   Yes [ ] No [X]

6. Is pregnant
   Yes [ ] No [X] N/A [ ]

MEDICAL HISTORY

She has experienced a recent weight loss of 10 lbs.

DENTAL HISTORY

This client receives regular dental care, breathes through her mouth and had orthodontic treatment in her early teens. She self-reports that she bites her fingernails.

SOCIAL HISTORY

As a full-time college student with a part-time job, this client is extremely busy and does not participate in a regular exercise regimen. Some of her meals are rushed and she is concerned about eating well-balanced meals.

CHIEF COMPLAINT

She has noticed that her gums look different and that they are sore and bleed. She is interested in having her teeth whitened.

ADULT CLINICAL EXAMINATION

Current oral hygiene status

This client presents with very slight calculus that is localized interproximally and slight generalized plaque in the interproximal areas.

Supplemental oral examination findings

Upon examination the following were noted:

1. Generalized moderate bleeding upon probing (BOP) in posterior regions
2. Localized slight BOP in maxillary anterior facial areas
3. Moderate xerostomia

Clinically visible carious lesion

Clinically missing tooth

△ Furcation

▲ "Through and through" furcation

Probe 1: Initial probing depth

Probe 2: Probing depth 3 months after scaling and root planing

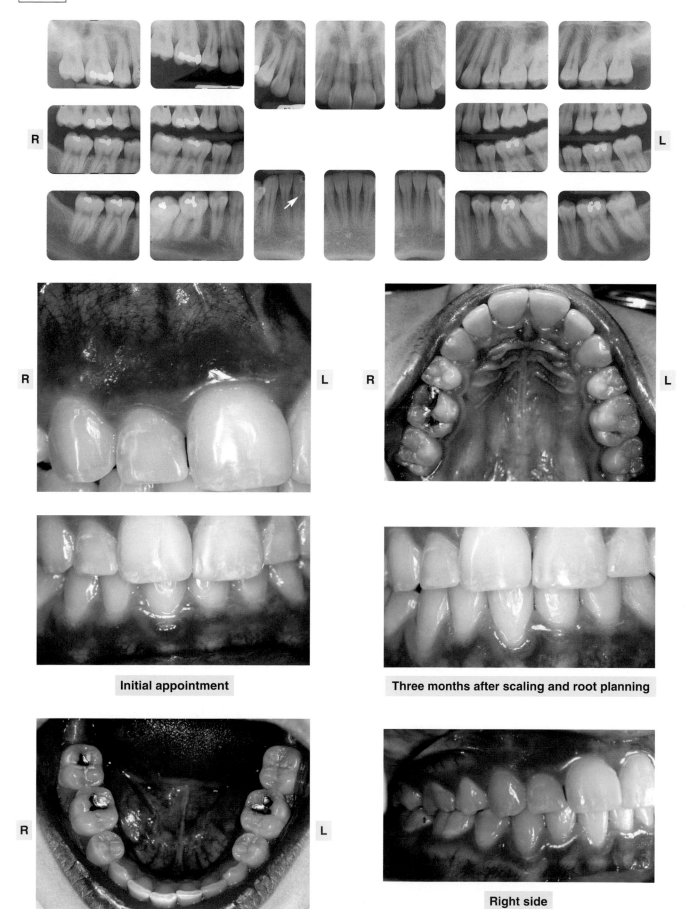

Initial appointment

Three months after scaling and root planning

Right side